CYCLING
Towards Health and Safet

The British Medical Association (BMA) is a professional organization representing all doctors in the UK. It was established in 1832 'to promote the medical and allied sciences, and to maintain the honour and interests of the medical profession'. The BMA Board of Science and Education supports this aim by providing an interface between the profession, the government, and the public, and by undertaking research studies on behalf of the Association. Through the publication of policy statements the Board of Science has led the debate on key public health issues.

The overriding objective of the Board of Science is to contribute to the development of better public health policies that affect the community, the state, and the medical profession. In order to do this, investigations need to be carried out by the Board on the impact of various policies and activities on the public health. The Board appoints working parties, combining medical and other specialist expertise, to carry out research on a variety of important issues. The Board has produced a large number of publications over recent years reflecting current concerns in the public health arena, such as alcohol and tobacco abuse, AIDS, nutrition, infection control, hazardous waste, and chemical pesticides.

Road traffic accidents and injuries have been a major concern of the British Medical Association for many years. In the past, the Association has taken a lead in examining road-safety issues such as seat belts, drink-driving, random breath testing, and general transport safety. The current work on cycling not only extends the Association's involvement in road safety but also the Board's interests in the wider issues of the environment and public health and the nature of risk in the natural and industrial world.

A report from the BMA
Professional, Scientific, and International Affairs Division

Project Director	Dr Fleur Fisher
Editor	David R. Morgan
Written by	Dr Mayer Hillman (Policy Studies Institute)
Contributors	Juliet Solomon
	Dr Ronald J. Maughan
	Josh Hillman
Editorial Secretariat	Sallie Robins
	Tara Lamont
Graphics	Hilary Glanville

CYCLING

Towards Health and Safety

BRITISH MEDICAL ASSOCIATION

Oxford   New York

OXFORD UNIVERSITY PRESS

1992

Oxford University Press, Walton Street, Oxford OX2 6DP

Oxford New York Toronto
Delhi Bombay Calcutta Madras Karachi
Petaling Jaya Singapore Hong Kong Tokyo
Nairobi Dar es Salaam Cape Town
Melbourne Auckland
and associated companies in
Berlin Ibadan

Oxford is a trade mark of Oxford University Press

First published 1992 as an Oxford University Press paperback
and simultaneously in a hardback edition

British Library Cataloguing in Publication Data
Data available

Library of Congress Cataloging in Publication Data
Cycling: towards health and safety / British Medical Association.
p.   cm.
Includes bibliographical references.
1. Cycling—Great Britain—Safety measures.   I. British Medical
Association.
GV1055.C93 1992   363.12'59—dc20   91–42620
ISBN 0–19–217783–4
ISBN 0–19–286151–4 (Pbk)

Text processed by Oxuniprint, Oxford University Press
Printed in Great Britain by
Richard Clay Ltd.
Bungay, Suffolk

CONTENTS

TABLES & FIGURES

Tables

Figures

ABBREVIATIONS

ATB	All-Terrain Bike
BMA	British Medical Association
BMX	Bicycle Moto-Cross
BST	British Summer Time
CTC	Cyclists' Touring Club
EC	European Community
GMT	Greenwich Mean Time
HEA	Health Education Authority
HDL	High-Density Lipoprotein
LASS	Leisure Accidents Surveillance System
LCC	London Cycling Campaign
LDL	Low-Density Lipoprotein
MAIS	Maximum Abbreviated Injury Scale
NCPS	National Cycling Proficiency Scheme
NHS	National Health Service
OPCS	Office of Population Censuses and Surveys
PE	Physical Education
RCN	Royal College of Nursing
RoSPA	Royal Society for the Prevention of Accidents
SMR	Standardized Mortality Ratios
TPPs	Transport Policies and Programmes
TRRL	Transport and Road Research Laboratory
UN	United Nations
VOC	Volatile Organic Compound
WHO	World Health Organization

Introduction

The bicycle is not a new invention, but over the past few years bicycles have enjoyed a new wave of popularity. New developments in cycle design, and new applications such as those made possible by BMX and mountain bikes, together with increased interest in health and fitness, have brought cycling as a leisure pursuit and means of transport to an increasing number of people.

Probably the earliest prototype of the bicycle appears among the manuscripts of Leonardo da Vinci, although this appears to have been a sketch made by a pupil using the technical ideas of his master. In spite of the Industrial Revolution's obsession with superseding the physical energy of humans and animals, no serious attempt was made at constructing a practical human-powered vehicle until the early part of the last century, when a craze developed in Europe and North America for a wheeled running machine or 'hobby-horse', usually a wooden contraption astride which people propelled themselves with their feet.

The only innovations that were made in the following few decades were extraordinary machines patented by amateur mechanics, for instance employing rotary or treadle-driven cranks. The major breakthrough came in France in the 1860s when the velocipede, or 'bone-shaker', with direct-drive pedals on the front wheel, was developed. It was used not only for amusement and racing, but also for commuting on a fairly large scale in Paris. Within a few years, it was frequently seen in many other European countries. In the US, more sophisticated models appeared on the market, with brakes and replaceable parts.

In Britain and the US in the 1880s, high bicycles or 'ordinarys', now known as penny-farthings, usually with tangential spokes and hubs containing ball-bearings—a highly significant technological break-through—became the standard model and formed the focus of attention for bicycle clubs. Their members were mainly middle-class city men who generally met once a week to participate in ritualistic rides, interspersed with a range of other activities such as dining, drinking, and gambling. Meanwhile, tricycles were developed and used by the upper classes and the 'respectable' professions, such as clergymen and doctors.

A decade later, low, rear-wheel-driven bicycles were replacing the high-wheel bicycle as the standard model. These 'safety' bicycles featured adjustable handlebars and seats, and sprung saddles. Most significantly, the pneumatic tyre was patented leading to further developments in cycling as a competitive sport. After the turn of the century, vast increases in productive efficiency and a burgeoning market allowed the cost of bicycles to fall sufficiently to allow working people of modest means to buy one. In Britain, cycling also became associated with the socialist movement, with the bicycle seen as the epitome of a compassionate and civilized way of life.

Since then, the basic design of the bicycle has not changed very much, although the derailleur gear reducing the need to dismount on hills, and the wide range of cycles with carriers allowing tradesmen to deliver goods to the home, were important innovations of the inter-war years. During this period cycling achieved its greatest popularity. However, the advent of the wider ownership of cars in the post-war years spelled a marked decline for cycling and its attractions because cars were seen to be a more comfortable and convenient form of transport. In addition, the ninefold increase in traffic since then has led to the decline in the quality and safety of the environment for cyclists. As a consequence, the number of miles cycled has declined dramatically. Government has done little to encourage local authorities to provide for cycling, but instead has focused its attention on promoting the ownership of cars and attempting to accommodate their use.

In recent years, cycling has grown in popularity, partly owing to the emergence of a new environmental consciousness. A rapidly increasing proportion of the population is choosing to cycle for leisure purposes,[1] and cycling is becoming more widely recognized again as a convenient, flexible, efficient, and fast means of travel on a door-to-door basis for journeys up to three to five miles—a fifteen- to thirty-minute ride. A daily cycle ride for twenty to thirty minutes covering a round trip of five miles as all or part of the journey to and from work can be quicker than travel by public transport and, in some areas, by car.[2] Cycling is thus able to compete effectively with motorized modes of transport on short journeys, especially those made by public transport which typically entail a walk at either end of the journey and a wait at the bus-stop. It is generally pleasurable, stress-free, and undoubtedly a very cheap form of travel, the main cost being the purchase-price. A bicycle costs approximately a fortieth as much as a family car, and with proper care and attention, it has a longer life. There are no fuel costs or taxes, insurance premiums are small, and cycles are relatively easy to maintain.

However, it is not simply the attractions of cycling to the individual that need to be considered. It offers an ideal solution to a wide range of current social, economic, and environmental problems. From the viewpoint of social justice, it should be borne in mind that nearly two in five households are non car-owning, and indeed the majority of people do not now have the optional use of a car. Even among adults, there are only about 20 million cars for the 40 million or so people who, in theory, fulfil the prerequisites for driving their own car, namely being old enough to do so, having adequate income, being physically capable, and having sufficient competence to drive. On the other hand, the great majority of the population—children as well as adults—can cycle. And for children, there is no other form of mechanized transport that they can use on their own.

In marked contrast to the car, use of the bicycle is unlikely to increase the risk of injury to other road-users. The bicycle does not need large areas of road or other resources when it is ridden or parked. The costs of making provision for people commuting by cycle are only a very small proportion of that for people commuting by car.[3] It contributes little to road congestion, taking up only about one-tenth of the space of a car, plus it adds nothing to traffic noise or pollution, which in combination have markedly lowered the amenity and quality of life.

A further benefit of cycling lies in the field of energy conservation. The consensus of scientific opinion now points to the need for dramatic reductions in the use of finite fossil fuels in order to lessen the damaging effects of carbon dioxide and other gases destabilizing the world's climate. For life on the planet to be sustainable in the long term, consumption of fossil fuels will need to be dramatically curtailed in all sectors of the economy. Fuel consumption for cycling is of course zero, while petrol consumption for car travel is responsible for a rising proportion of greenhouse gases.

It is also important to bear in mind that current patterns of petrol consumption will soon have the effect of significantly adding to the country's dependence upon imported oil once our indigenous reserves in the North Sea have been used up. Some measure of the contribution that cycling makes today to fuel conservation can be appreciated from the fact that if everyone who currently makes their journeys by bicycle were to travel by car, at typical levels of car occupancy, it would lead to a national increase of 2 per cent of the 7,000 million gallons of petrol that cars use each year.[4]

These considerations represent substantial grounds for planning a more significant role for cycling in future patterns of transport, and point to society's interests being well served if more people were enabled and encouraged to use bicycles on a regular basis. Further grounds for doing so have been suggested recently in view of the very strong links between transport and health. The need has been recognized for interaction not only between the two government departments with responsibility for these two domains of policy, but also interaction with the wide range of other departments, such as environment, energy, and education, the policies of which indirectly influence decisions on transport and health.[5]

In 1990, a conference which dealt exclusively with cycling and health raised a wide range of issues relevant to the evolution of progressive policies reflecting the considerable scope that cycling may have in health promotion.[6] Such issues should become of increasing importance in the light of the Government's consultative document, *The Health of the Nation*, which gives targets for improved levels of national health and fitness and also for reducing road traffic accidents.[7]

Why is cycling of interest to the medical profession?

Doctors have an interest in cycling for two reasons: first, the alarmingly high rate of fatal and serious accidents suffered by cyclists, and secondly, the role that cycling has to play in preventing ill health in the community as a whole. In this sense, cycling can be seen as a concern of wider public-health interests.

Indeed, it was the concern of the medical profession over the high levels of death and injury to cyclists that led to debate of the subject at the 1989 British Medical Association (BMA) Annual Representatives Meeting (ARM). A resolution was passed calling upon the Association to investigate measures to effect improvements in the safety of cyclists in view of the continuing high level of death and injury among cyclists involved in road-traffic accidents. As a result of this debate the Board of Science and Education was asked to set up a steering group and produce a report examining the physiology, psychology, and health benefits associated with cycling and the morbidity and mortality associated with bicycle use. The Board was also asked to investigate the pattern of bicycle usage and current safety provisions in the UK and other countries, to assess the safety of cyclists and make recommendations as to how this can be improved.

Road-traffic accidents and the number of fatalities have been a major concern of the BMA for many years. In the past, the Association has taken a lead in examining road-safety issues such as seat-belts, drink-driving, random breath-testing, and general transport safety; such involvement has now been extended to include this extensive review of cycling. Mechanisms to improve the safety of cyclists, such as a reduction in urban motor-vehicle speeds, will also affect the overall safety of *all* road users and may make a significant contribution to lowering the high number of people killed on the roads every year.

As a professional and scientific body, the BMA is concerned with the wider issues of environmental and public health, prompting previous investigations into alcohol and tobacco abuse, and the nature of risk in the natural and industrial worlds. Cycling contributes to the public health not only through the beneficial effects to the individual of taking this form of aerobic exercise, but also to the wider public health through the reduction in air pollution from motor vehicles that would result from an increase in cycle use as a serious means of city transportation.

What is the scope of the report?

This report is not intended to be a practical guide to those who currently cycle, or who wish to take up cycling. Rather it attempts to review the current situation for cyclists in the UK, particularly in relation to the risk faced on our increasingly hazardous roads, and to consider the part that regular exercise can play in improving health, in particular the specific advantages of cycling as a form of exercise.

Chapter 2 looks at the health-benefits of cycling as a regular means of aerobic exercise. The general benefits of taking regular exercise are examined in the context of the current state of the nation's health. The chapter looks at both the physiological and psychological benefits of exercise. Lung and respiratory function, cardiovascular disease, obesity, and mental health are identified as areas in which exercise may have a particular role.

Chapter 3 investigates current patterns of cycle ownership and use. Although there is evidence that cycle sales are increasing and that the great majority of the population can cycle, it only plays a very small role in current patterns of travel. The changing role that cycling has played in travel-patterns over the past century is also examined.

Chapter 4 discusses the reasons for the low use of bicycles compared to the high levels of ownership. In particular, the chapter examines the deterrent effects of effort, climate, cycle theft, work-environment, and attitudes. The two major issues of road safety and air pollution, due to their central role in the debate, are examined in depth in following chapters.

Chapter 5 examines the issue of paramount importance to those concerned with cycling policy and promotion: the safety of cyclists on the road. Available statistics are presented and the reasons for the unreliability of much of the data explained. The relative importance of different factors creating hazards for cyclists is explored. An analysis is also made of the estimated costs of accidents involving cyclists in order that the cost-effectiveness of improved provision for this particular type of road-user can be demonstrated.

Chapter 6 outlines the effects of air pollution on the cyclist, the general population, and the environment. The short-term effects of breathing car-exhaust fumes and the long-term effects on the environment are discussed, with acknowledgement of the difficulties of measuring the effects of pollution on health. The contribution that cycling could make to reductions in levels of air pollution is also examined.

Chapter 7 attempts to estimate the latent demand for cycling based on levels of cycle-ownership and current conditions for cyclists on UK roads. The chapter examines the potential that cycling may have in catering for a much higher proportion of journeys. Cycle use in the UK is compared with that in other European countries in order that the reasons for the low levels of usage in this country can be determined.

Chapter 8 presents the arguments regarding the role of the individual in countering some of the risks of cycling. The somewhat controversial issue of protective headgear is reviewed, with the debate regarding legislation to make cycle helmets compulsory fully explored. Also discussed is the role that child-cyclist training, conspicuity aids, and pollution masks can play in protecting the cyclist. Throughout the chapter, the central question of who should carry responsibility for the safety of cyclists is discussed.

Chapter 9 reviews current policy on cycling and provides a discussion basis for future policy directions in planning and provision for cycling. The experience of other European countries is reviewed in order to determine mechanisms by which cycling can be promoted as a serious means of transportation. Public attitudes towards cycling are also considered in their context as a barrier to the wider use of cycles.

Chapter 10 seeks to weigh up the disadvantages of cycling stemming from its relatively high casualty-rate with the benefits in terms of its health-promoting properties. Data on estimated life-years gained due to the improved health of regular cyclists are presented alongside data on estimated number of life-years lost through accidents.

This report was prepared under the auspices of the Board of Science and Education of the British Medical Association. The members of the Board were as follows:

Professor A. C. Kennedy	*President, BMA*
Dr A. Macara	*Chairman, Representative Body, BMA*
Dr J. Lee-Potter	*Chairman, BMA Council*
Dr J. A. Riddell	*Treasurer, BMA*
Professor J. B. L. Howell	*Chairman, Board of Science and Education*
Professor J. P. Payne	*Deputy Chairman, Board of Science*
Dr J. M. Cundy	
Dr A. Elliott	
Dr R. Farrow	
Dr M. Goodman	
Dr L. P. Grime	
Dr D. Milne	
Dr G. M. Mitchell	
Col. M. J. G. Thomas L/RAMC	
Dr D. Ward	

A Steering Group with the following membership was set up in order to provide expert guidance:

Mr P. Bewes	*Consultant Surgeon, Department of Surgery, Birmingham Accident Hospital*
Mr K. Clinton	*National Cycling Officer, Royal Society for the Prevention of Accidents*
Dr J. Cundy	*Member, Board of Science and Education; Consultant Anaesthetist, Lewisham Hospital*
Mr H. McClintock	*Lecturer, Institute of Planning Studies, University of Nottingham; database compiler for the Local Authorities Cycle Planning Group; Chairman of 'Pedals' (Nottingham Cycling Campaign)*
Ms J. Renfree	*Research Officer, Cambridge Project on the Psychology of Cycling, Hughes Hall, Cambridge*

Mr R. Wakeford   *Director, Cambridge Project on the Psychology of Cycling, Hughes Hall, Cambridge*

Further expert advice was provided by: Mr D. Mathew, Dr R. J. Maughan, Dr J. R. Sibert, Mr A. Fowler, Dr M. McCarthy, Dr C. Bannister, Dr J. Gosnold, Mr W. Tuxworth.

European advisers: Mr Jan Ploeger (Consultant on Cycling Safety for the ENFB Cyclists' Association, Delft, the Netherlands), Mr André Pettinga (Transportation Planner and Traffic Engineer, State Company for Road Provision, Delft, the Netherlands), Mr Tom Godefrooij (Policy Co-ordinator for the ENFB Cyclists' Association, Woerden, the Netherlands), Ms Ingrid van Schagen (Traffic Research Centre, University of Gröningen, the Netherlands).

CHAPTER TWO

The health-and-fitness benefits of cycling

This chapter examines the health-and-fitness aspects of cycling, perhaps the least-researched area of policy on cycling although it may provide the most compelling reasons for encouraging participation. It explores some of the general effects of physical exercise, and reports on the growing body of evidence that links regular exercise to improved health. It describes various common causes of morbidity and mortality, and sees how far increased levels of exercise are considered to be either preventative or therapeutic. Subsequently, the contribution that cycling could make to improving the health of the nation is discussed.

The educational system in Greece in classical times included gymnastics, as well as mathematics and music, as essential daily activities, and the Romans coined the motto 'Mens sana in corpore sano'—a healthy mind in a healthy body. The inclusion of physical activity in the school curriculum was a clear recognition of the link between regular exercise and health. Since then, the association between physical fitness and health has been more closely investigated and the virtues of maintaining fitness in all its manifestations have been almost universally recognized. Nevertheless, Britain's population still contains a high proportion of people who are neither fit nor healthy. The lifestyle that has been developing during this century is one of increasing sedentariness in most respects. At work, the proportion of people employed in non-manual occupations increased from 30 per cent in 1931 to 52 per cent in 1981, and has risen sharply since then.[1] In the home, too, the amount of housework which involves hard physical effort has decreased substantially as more labour-saving devices have been introduced. Even office jobs now involve less effort—with very little movement of individuals being required for communication with colleagues.

The journey to work which, in the earlier part of this century might quite commonly have involved walking several miles a day, may now require no more exertion than stepping out from home into a car, sometimes with power-assisted steering, being dropped at a station whose stairs have been replaced by an escalator, sitting in a train, and walking a hundred yards before getting into a lift in an office-building. Exercise, which was once an integral part of daily life from early child-hood onwards, has now become for many people a consciously sought-out leisure activity. More typically, it has been avoided as part of the instinctive urge to minimize effort.[2] Routine physical exercise has also been reduced among children. Four times as many junior schoolchildren are now taken to school by car as were taken twenty years ago.[3] Once skipping, playing on the streets, and going for bicy-cle rides were indulged in quite spontaneously by children. For a mul-tiplicity of reasons these activities are now much less common, their place having largely been taken by the passive leisure pursuit of tele-vision viewing.

At present, the fitness and health of the nation is difficult to monitor as, regrettably, there is no regular national survey of such key ele-ments as changes in physical performance. However, the occasional 'snapshot' suggests that only a small proportion of adults get sufficient exercise to maintain their fitness. The findings from the Na-tional Travel Surveys conducted during the 1970s and 1980s indicate that walking, a very convenient form of regular exercise, is declining as a travel method.[4] Whilst there has been a minor renaissance in cy-cling in the last few years, cycling only accounts for 3 per cent of all personal journeys and 1 per cent of all personal mileage.[5]

In the face of the increasing transfer towards more mechanized and sedentary life-styles, it would be reassuring if this did not incur some cost for society. However, research findings over the last few decades have established the benefits to health of improving physical con-dition through the medium of fairly vigorous and regular physical ex-ercise. These benefits are now widely cited by proprietors of increasing numbers of health-centres and health-farms, and manu-facturers of exercise machines, as well as by organizations such as the

Health Education Authority which are active in the field of health promotion.

The link between habitual physical activity and physical fitness is obvious, and it is equally clear that the training response is specific to the training activity. Lifting heavy loads increases muscle mass and develops strength, whereas endurance is developed by prolonged, relatively low-intensity, rhythmic activities such as swimming, walking, or cycling. The association between regular exercise and health, although less immediately apparent, is no less real. The distinction between fitness and health is often blurred, and indeed the two, although not inseparable, are closely related.

A definition of these two concepts might be useful. Fitness relates to the ability to carry out a specific task. We usually think of physical fitness in relation to sports performance, but it has important implications for the whole population and for everyday tasks. While muscle strength is most highly developed in the weight-lifter, some degree of muscular strength is important for everyone. For example, the quadriceps muscle, which extends the knee and hip, is used in most daily activities such as walking, stair-climbing, and in moving from a sitting to a standing position. Because of this regular exercise it is usually strong enough to cope with the demands placed upon it. With age, however, activity-levels generally decrease and some degree of muscle-wasting and loss of strength occur; with immobilization or bed-rest this process is greatly accelerated. If an individual's muscle strength decreases to the point where it is less than that necessary to lift the body from a sitting to a standing position, then independence is lost—that person will no longer be able to climb stairs or go to the toilet unaided.

Endurance fitness is no less important in maintaining the quality of life. While relatively few people want to run a marathon, a reasonable level of fitness makes it possible to cope with the physical demands of everyday life without undue stress. It is also important in maintaining mobility and independence, and allows us to walk or play football with our children and grandchildren.

Health is more difficult to define, and is often described as an absence of illness, but health should be more than this and should involve a feeling of positive well-being. Improvements in the health of the general population are associated with a reduction in morbidity and an increased longevity.

The following range of beneficial effects on health and fitness have been described by the Coronary Prevention Group:[6]

FITNESS

- Increase in maximal oxygen uptake and cardiac output/stroke volume
- Reduced heart-rate at a given oxygen uptake
- Reduced heart-rate at rest
- Improved efficiency of heart muscle
- Increased capillary density in skeletal muscle
- Increased activity of aerobic enzymes in skeletal muscles
- Reduced lactate production at given levels of oxygen uptake
- Enhanced ability to utilize free fatty acid during exercise
- Improved endurance
- Improved strength of muscles, ligaments, tendons, and bones
- Reduced perceived effort at a given work-rate
- Enhanced tolerance of high temperatures through increased sweating

HEALTH

- Reduced cardiac morbidity and mortality
- Increased metabolic rate with advantages from a nutritional viewpoint
- An antidote to obesity
- An increase in the HDL/LDL ratio
- Decreased blood pressure
- Delayed onset of post-menopausal osteoporosis
- Improved glucose tolerance in diabetes
- Possible improvements in mental health

Obviously there is some degree of overlap between these effects. The reduced rate of coronary disease among those who exercise on a regular basis is probably closely related to the effects of exercise in reducing body fat, in reducing blood pressure in hypertensive individuals, and in altering the blood-cholesterol profile. With so many benefits, it is not surprising that a correlation between physical activity and mortality has been established. A major study in the US involving monitoring 13,000 people over several years recorded a substantial difference between the fit and the unfit. The study concluded that: 'higher levels of physical fitness appear to delay all-cause mortality, primarily due to lowered rates of cardiovascular disease and cancer.'[7] This study provided clear evidence that, even though the process is not wholly understood, exercise in moderation does contribute to reducing the risk of premature death.

Why should exercise be so beneficial? The intuitive answer can be found in the observation that the human body is designed for movement. To develop and maintain peak levels of physical fitness, exercise must be carried out on a regular basis and must be relatively strenuous. For the sedentary individual, sudden, strenuous movements are inadvisable and can be dangerous. Adequate levels of fitness will, however, result from rather modest amounts of exercise. The recommended amount of exercise from a health perspective is about twenty to thirty minutes of moderate exercise three times a week. The level of activity which produces a benefit is related to the initial level of fitness: for the middle-aged sedentary individual, this may correspond to walking, cycling slowly, or gentle swimming.

The energy which is needed for exercise comes from two major series of chemical reactions, anaerobic and aerobic. In anaerobic exercise, energy is released by the muscles without the involvement of oxygen: although the chemical reactions involved release energy rapidly, they have a limited capacity and fatigue sets in quickly. The end-product of these reactions is lactic acid, and when this accumulates within the muscle further exercise will not be possible. Anaerobic work is carried out during high-intensity exercise when the demand for energy exceeds that which can be met by aerobic metabolism: some anaerobic-energy release also occurs at the onset of exercise as the delivery of oxygen to the muscle increases only slowly. During aerobic exercise, oxygen remains available to the muscle for continuing efficient, energy-yielding reactions, and the exercise can thus be sustained over a much longer period.

Aerobic exercise is increasingly recognized as being of primary importance in producing the health-related benefits associated with physical activity. These include general fitness, muscle-strength and flexibility, improved lung-and-heart functioning, increased bone formation and maintenance of bone-mass, control of body-weight, and reduction of obesity and improved mental health.

General fitness

Muscular tissue is extremely plastic: it is developed by exercise, and deteriorates if not used. Adaptations to exercise can be seen within a few days, and disuse will result in an equally rapid reversal of functional capacity. An insufficiency of movement over a prolonged period, such as occurs during immobilization after injury or during bed-rest, will result in tissue-degeneration and eventually in malfunction. In general, the body's tissues respond and adapt themselves to the stresses imposed upon them, but they do need some stress. The strengthening of this tissue comes through the use of specific muscles—that is, the training response occurs only in those muscles which are used.

Muscle-endurance and strength develop from early childhood, but recent studies have shown that suitable training will result in gains in muscle-strength even in extreme old age. The need for maintaining an adequate level of muscle-strength to permit an independent lifestyle has already been mentioned. Inactivity and muscle-weakness may also be associated with a variety of other problems, including an increase in hip fracture—a common problem among the elderly, as discussed later. Clearly the major muscles associated with the movement of limbs are worth preserving in good condition for as long as possible.[8]

There are many kinds of exercise which develop and encourage the use of specific muscles and bring about an improvement in general muscle-tone. Swimming is undoubtedly an ideal exercise for developing stamina, strength, and flexibility, as virtually all muscles are used in unstressed movements. Some kinds of dancing also have these characteristics. However, in all these cases difficulties arise owing to the costs and problems of access to facilities. Paying entry-charges several times a week can be prohibitive, particularly if transport-costs such as bus-fares have to be added. Moreover, the average public swimming-pool serves a population of over 45,000 people, posing prospects of severe congestion in the pool if only 1 per cent were to swim regularly.

Aerobics has the same problems of cost and restricted access. Jogging and running are convenient and relatively inexpensive activities, but have a limited appeal to most individuals. Although they have enjoyed a considerable increase in popularity in recent years, it is unlikely that they will ever involve more than a small fraction of the population.

Cycling is more limited than these forms of exercise in the actual variety of muscles which are exercised. However, it has 'built-in' rest periods between its submaximal rhythms which make long spells easier and reduce anaerobic elements, fatigue, and lactic-acid accumulation. Furthermore, there are obvious advantages to cycling as a form of fitness training. It can be undertaken regularly by people of all ages and as a part of daily life, without specific facilities being called for (except safer streets), and with little risk of injury from 'overuse'. It is potentially one of the most appropriate ways for individuals to maintain their fitness through the rhythmic contraction and relaxation of the large limb muscles.[9] In contrast to running and jogging, which can place high stress on hips, knees, ankles, and the Achilles tendons, there is very little risk of cycling leading to overstrain of muscles, ligaments, or other injuries from 'overuse', particularly as the body is supported on a saddle, with pressure and effort distributed between two hands, two feet, and one backside.

Lung and respiratory function

The requirement of the working muscles for oxygen and the adaptations in the cardio-respiratory system and within the muscles themselves are the keys to an understanding of the role of exercise. There is a direct relationship between the amount of oxygen taken up by the body and the intensity of an exercise task. For each individual, there is an upper limit to the rate of oxygen uptake which can be achieved when exercising, and this is the most important determinant of endurance performance, though it can be improved. When it is, not only is the limit raised, but so is the amount of time that activity below the limit can be sustained.[10] The limit to oxygen uptake is normally set by the ability of the heart to deliver oxygen-rich blood to the working muscles.

Adequate respiratory function is essential for good health. It is a composite of the purely mechanical process of breathing and the ability of the heart and the blood to transport oxygen to the tissues and carbon dioxide back to the lungs. It is clear that vigorous exercise, which increases deep breathing, involves the lungs in taking in more oxygen and dispelling more carbon dioxide than when at rest. Regular exercise stimulates the use of breathing muscles which then respond to this training-load in the same way that other muscles do. Changes in the lungs themselves are minimal, but training does improve the delivery of oxygen to respiratory muscles.[11]

Breathing exercises have been prescribed for years in patients with chronic conditions, such as asthma and bronchitis. While sufferers from asthma have to be careful when exercising,[12] it does appear that some exercise can have a beneficial effect in extending their capacity for exertion. Moderately vigorous cycling is therefore a suitable way of doing this. An important caveat to this, discussed more fully in a later chapter, is that those with respiratory problems should avoid cycling in areas with high levels of air pollution.[13]

Cardiovascular disease

Diseases of the heart and circulation ('cardiovascular diseases'), together with cancer, are the commonest causes of death in Britain. Coronary heart disease accounts for about 80 per cent of heart disease and is the greatest single cause of death, being responsible for a third of all deaths in men and a quarter in women. It has been calculated that treatment of heart-related conditions cost the NHS over £500 million in 1988, but this figure only accounts for direct medical expenses. Added to this are the costs associated with time off work, which have been estimated at 41.5 million working days at a cost to industry of £1.8 billion.[14] There are also unquantifiable costs in terms of personal and family anxiety, limitation of activity, and so on.[15]

The heart pumps blood round the system, taking oxygen to various parts of the body. The ease with which the heart can carry out this task determines the amount of strain it experiences. About 70 ml of blood is pumped with each of the heart's daily 100,000 beats, which for the average individual works out at about five litres a minute at rest. During vigorous exercise, blood-flow can increase to 25 litres a minute. This increased blood-flow enables more oxygen to be delivered to tissues, with most of it going to the exercising muscles.[16]

The factors which are now most commonly understood to be associated with coronary heart disease are high cholesterol levels, raised blood pressure, smoking, obesity, and stress. Cholesterol can be broadly divided into the 'good' type, HDL (high-density lipoprotein), and the 'bad' type, LDL (low-density lipoprotein). The higher the ratio of HDL to LDL, the more likely the heart and its coronary arteries are to be healthy. If the ratio is low, cholesterol can get deposited on the walls of the arteries causing them to fur up (atherosclerosis), resulting in reduced flow of blood. High levels of HDL cholesterol can help to remove some of the cholesterol from artery walls and transport it to the liver where it is metabolized. Many studies have shown that exercise leads to changes in the proportions of high- and low-density lipoproteins which should reduce the incidence of both atherosclerosis and coronary thrombosis: the level of LDL is decreased and the level of HDL is increased in response to training.[17]

Blood itself must always be under some pressure to circulate, but if the pressure rises too high the heart has to work harder, again increasing the risk of coronary problems.[18] Regular exercise can lead to a fall in blood pressure when this is already higher than normal, and is potentially a major non-pharmacological method of lowering blood pressure.[19] Insurance statistics show that men with only moderately high blood pressure (hypertension) can expect to live about fifteen years less than men with low blood pressure.[20] Obesity, which is discussed later, is a further contributory factor, albeit indirect, in that it has adverse effects both on cholesterol levels and blood pressure.

Stress is difficult to define. It is required to a certain extent for healthy functioning. Studies have not been able to show precisely what role it plays in heart disease, but it is known that stress produces adrenaline, which stimulates the heart to beat faster. Under too much stress blood pressure rises, the rate of blood coagulation increases and the liver releases sugar and fats into the bloodstream to provide energy. An increase in the blood-coagulation rate increases the chances of blood-clots, and the excess fat in the blood can be deposited in the arteries. Temporary stress (like anything else in moderation) appears not to be a problem—the body simply readjusts until the stress is over—but if it is persistent the system becomes overloaded.[21]

Until fairly recently, people with heart conditions were often told to rest as a cure. However, the role of physical activity and inactivity in causing and in treating coronary heart disease has been the subject of a considerable body of research. Some of the earliest work was carried out in Britain nearly forty years ago and involved a comparative study of bus drivers and bus conductors.[22] The incidence of coronary disease was higher among the drivers, who were sedentary, than among the more-active conductors. Since then the relevance of this issue has come increasingly to the fore. Further research over the years has confirmed the major preventive role that daily exercise can play in lowering the incidence of this disease.[23] Men whose work or leisure activities involve vigorous exercise are less likely than their non-exercising contemporaries to develop or die of coronary heart disease. Several of these studies, particularly those from North America, have suggested that only rather low levels of activity are necessary to confer some degree of protection against heart disease, both in terms of the intensity of effort and of the total amount of exercise taken.

Although medical science has made much progress in the understanding of the causes of heart disease and in the efficacy of various forms of treatment, knowledge is still incomplete. Nevertheless, there is now a considerable body of evidence to support the view that death from this disease is often preventable.

Life-cycle and the heart

Although, as a preventive measure, the prescription for adults of vigorous exercise for at least twenty minutes three times a week is now broadly acknowledged,[24] it is not clear at what age this should start, nor, in view of changing physiological demands, what level of activity is required at each stage of the life-cycle for hearts to function optimally. However, there is some consensus that the prescription for children would not be dissimilar to that for adults.

Surveys have shown that primary schoolchildren are not sufficiently active to maintain a reasonable level of fitness.[25] A second study found that 15-year-old girls were less fit than 50-year-old men.[26] A third, carried out to determine how much exercise was taken by British schoolchildren aged 11 to 16, has shown levels of habitual physical activity to be surprisingly low.[27] It suggested that part of the problem lies with children's attitudes and motivations, and that there is a need to make exercise more fun.

The issue of children's exercise is crucial not only because of its link with their health and fitness in later life, but also because habits such as taking part in and enjoying physical activity are most easily acquired in childhood and may be difficult to acquire later. At the other end of the life-cycle, evidence suggests that exercise has a beneficial effect on the heart even if it is taken up late in life, and that in fact a therapeutic effect can be achieved with a more leisurely level of exercise than that required by younger people.[28]

Why cycling for the heart?

It is clear, both from epidemiological and clinical studies, that exercise is likely to benefit the heart. The exercise that is most frequently suggested is brisk walking—ordinary strolling appears to have little effect. Swimming, tennis, and various other active sports as well as cycling are also often recommended. Each of these activities has its own particular advantages and disadvantages. However, the attractions of cycling are many. First, as noted, it involves the rhythmic contraction of large limb muscles, and is therefore an ideal aerobic exercise. Secondly, even the gentlest cycling is a more strenuous exercise than is usual for a sedentary population, without the strain on muscles and joints associated with weight-bearing exercises. This may be particularly relevant to the overweight. Thirdly, it is a form of exercise that is easily available to most adults and children.

A sense of purpose often contributes to making an activity enjoyable. The use of bicycles, for instance in travelling to work, can provide this purpose, as long as safe provision is made for cyclists. Without such provision, the risk of injury when cycling may outweigh its positive cardiac-fitness benefits. However, a cautionary note needs to be sounded about people with coronary artery disease, who are particularly advised to avoid heavily trafficked city streets because of the dangers of breathing high levels of carbon monoxide, which is a contributory factor in cardiac arrhythmias.[29]

Direct evidence relating cycling *per se* to reduced rates of coronary heart disease is sparse, but several related studies can be mentioned. The first is the major longitudinal study referred to earlier,[30] which recorded that the small proportion of respondents who regularly cycled had a low incidence of this disease. However, it needs to be borne in mind that the association may be explained by the fact that the cyclists in the sample were healthy people because they were persuaded of the benefits of cycling and therefore encouraged to cycle. A short paper published in the *British Medical Journal* which looked specifically at cyclists, showed that there was a decrease in the incidence of myocardial infarction and ischaemic heart disease in all the cyclists studied, and a tenfold decrease in the incidence of ischaemic heart disease in the over-75 group.[31]

Another study, not specifically aimed at cycling, took a group of patients with heart problems and tested the effects on their heart of exercise on a bicycle machine which, although static, provides the same sort of exercise as cycling on the road. It concluded that: 'home-based physical training programmes are feasible even in severe chronic heart failure and have a beneficial effect on exercise tolerance, peak oxygen consumption, and symptoms. The commonly-held belief that rest is the mainstay of treatment of chronic heart failure should no longer be accepted.'[32]

Obesity

Medical evidence shows that obesity is a health-hazard. It exacerbates the effects of much morbidity, and is particularly associated with a greater likelihood of developing heart disease, hypertension, late-onset diabetes, arthritis, and bronchitis. It also increases the risk of complications during surgery. It is for this reason that life-insurance underwriters sometimes charge increased premiums for overweight people: according to their calculations, 7 per cent of the adult population in this country are seriously obese, that is, more than 30 per cent above a desirable height/weight ratio.[33] Moreover, a government survey has found that more than one in three adults in this country are overweight.[34]

There has been some controversy about the value of exercise in weight reduction. For instance, it has been established that it would be necessary to walk about thirty miles to use up the calories to burn off a pound of fat. However, if obese people maintain a constant calorie intake but walk or cycle a mile or two each day, they would end up considerably lighter at the end of the year.[35]

About four to five calories a minute are expended when cycling gently, that is three to four times higher than when a person is sitting at rest. Thus, cycling for half an hour a day uses 120 to 150 calories; on a routine five-day a week basis, up to 750 calories; and over a year, up to 40,000 calories. As the energy-value of one kilogram of adipose tissue is about 7,700 calories, cycling for half an hour a day expends an annual amount of energy equivalent to that stored in over five kilograms of adipose tissue. Individuals who undertake this amount of exercise but who are not overweight can eat rather more and can enjoy a more varied diet without an increase in body-fat content.

However, it is not only the actual calories burnt up that justifies exercise as part of an obesity-reducing regimen. If people simply eat fewer calories, their body's metabolic rate will slow down to compensate for the reduced intake, and weight-loss through dieting alone is an extremely slow process. Low energy intakes for prolonged periods also carry some risk of leading to specific nutritional deficiencies. The individual with a high energy intake will also have a high intake of vitamins, minerals, and trace elements. Strenuous exercise may also help to maintain a high metabolic rate for as much as twenty-four hours after the exercise itself. This suggests that regular exercise, taken as a part of the routine of daily life, is far more beneficial to the obese than is indicated simply by taking into account the energy expended.[36]

It is also worth noting that the risk of heart attack and other obesity-related illness can be reduced by exercise even among those who remain overweight. Obese people who exercise regularly have been found to have a risk of suffering a heart attack no greater than normal exercisers, whereas sedentary obese people have five times the risk.[37]

In the case of people who are simply overweight, that is, sub-clinical obesity which affects over a third of the population, particularly in middle-age, acquiring the habit of regular exercise not only helps to reduce weight, but also reduces the occurrence of heart attacks.

Obesity is not confined to the adult population. It can start in childhood, where it causes social as well as physical problems. Many, but not all, pre-pubertal children appear to enjoy physical activity and, even without encouragement, take sufficient exercise to derive the health-related benefits. However, as noted earlier, activity levels fall considerably during adolescence, especially among girls. A survey on this has recorded a fall in the average weekly time spent in PE (physical education) by 14-year-olds.[38] Published figures based on time allowed in the curriculum for physical activity will be an overestimate. In terms of active exercise time this is probably reduced by between a third and a half owing to changing, showering, and hanging about. Even that period of time could diminish owing to the pressures under the National Curriculum to cover what are considered by the education authorities to be more important subjects.

Games and PE periods in school have not been universally popular activities among adolescents, especially girls. When fewer households owned cars, more exercise was taken either by walking or cycling in the course of just getting about. Recreational activity is therefore more important than before, and some thought must be given to making it more attractive to youngsters. It could be inferred from the earlier discussion of metabolism that the previous generation of children had greater metabolic protection against obesity than has the more-sedentary current generation, which is therefore more dependent on diet to keep weight down during a period when a balanced diet is particularly important for their development.

Other health benefits of exercise

Habitual vigorous physical exercise not only has a significant preventive role for pulmonary and cardiovascular disease and obesity, it can also be beneficial in helping to reverse these conditions if they have already developed. Even if it had no other benefits, that would provide much justification for promoting exercise as part of the routine of daily life from an early age and for maintaining it throughout life. There are, however, also some beneficial effects for a range of other medical conditions.

Osteoporosis is a condition resulting from an increased porosity of the bones which allows them to fracture more easily. In spite of remarkable advances in surgery for the treatment of hip fractures, this condition still severely limits the independent mobility of many older women. Spinal osteoporosis can lead to collapse of the vertebrae, and to deformity and loss of height.

Whilst new hormone-replacement therapies have been found to be successful in combating the condition and in lowering the rising costs to the NHS for treatment of conditions such as hip fracture resulting from it, there is evidence that weight-bearing and muscle-loading exercise provide some protection. Physical activity and its attendant mechanical stresses stimulate bone metabolism, increasing bone-mass even after the menopause.[39] Osteoporosis has considerable socio-economic consequences in Western society. By the age of 70 about 40 per cent of women have experienced a fracture, resulting in a considerable economic burden on the Health Service.[40]

Cycling is not primarily a weight-bearing exercise, as the body is partly supported; local fatigue and excessive static loads on joints, muscles, and tendons is therefore avoided, which is important for the elderly or overweight. There is a degree of weight-bearing activity in cycling which provides some protection against osteoporosis of the arms. Protection against osteoporosis for the hips and legs is minimal, as there is very little weight-bearing within these areas. Nevertheless, cycling can provide some protection from fractures as the increased muscular strength gained from regular cycling means that an individual is less likely to fall and hence risk fractures.

Exercise may also help with the control of diabetes, as rhythmic exercise increases the sensitivity of body tissues to insulin. Therefore, physical training should be a highly effective and rational treatment for overweight, type 2 diabetic patients suffering from insulin resistance, hyperlipoproteinaemia, and often raised blood pressure.[41] Type 1 diabetic patients have a different problem, and the conditions under which exercise might benefit them are so specific that exercise would be unlikely to be particularly beneficial. Although the mechanisms by which exercise can help this condition are known, there has so far been no controlled study aimed at providing direct proof of its benefits.

Most exercise-and-health research concentrates on men, though some attention has been paid to women. Test results on pregnant women found that a group cycling or taking similar types of exercise for one hour, three times a week, at 85 per cent intensity, improved their cardiovascular fitness compared to controls who remained mostly sedentary. It has also been suggested that a high level of fitness may ease childbirth.[42]

Mental health

While it is established that regular exercise results in physiological benefits of various kinds, the benefits to mental health are harder to evaluate and are less well documented. A considerable amount of research is now being done on this issue, and the question of whether the psychological benefits of exercise can be demonstrated beyond anecdote has been discussed in medical and sports circles.[43] A major review of the subject drew three relevant conclusions: first, that there is evidence for both acute and long-term changes in brain monoamine turnover with exercise, although this link between exercise and alterations in mood is highly speculative; secondly, that there may be acute but not chronic changes in opioid peptides in the brain with exercise; and thirdly, that the benefits of exercise on depression may occur as a result of social interaction rather than any specific physiological effect.[44]

An experiment with individualized exercise programmes, thereby ruling out the possibility of social interaction being the explanation for any change observed, did, however, establish that regular aerobic exercise could significantly decrease depression.[45] This suggests that it is not only biochemical changes which help, but perhaps also improvements in confidence and self-esteem. It was also found that the benefits noted at the end of an eight-week exercise programme were maintained twenty weeks later for those subjects who continued with the programme. Another study of four population-surveys has indicated that exercise has a beneficial effect on depression and anxiety states.[46]

Evidence has been found of a link between endorphins—substances produced by the brain with a calming effect—and exercise.[47] Research has suggested that stimulating the body helps the brain to release endorphins, which can lift mood in the same way as helpful psychoactive drugs can. It has been suggested that aerobic exercise may be as good as drug therapy in mild to moderate cases of depression, even if the effects are sometimes short-term.[48] Indeed, habitual runners temporarily deprived of their routine were found to have significantly more symptoms of depression and anxiety after two weeks until they resumed running.[49] However, the link is acknowledged to be rather tenuous, owing to difficulties of interpretation of measurements made on blood-levels of substances that act on cells in the central nervous system.

Whether changes in mood as a result of exercise are physically or psychologically caused is hard to define, partly because the two are ultimately inseparable. As well as enhancing mood, aerobic exercise may be beneficial in reducing mental stress in general, in the sense that it raises tolerance to stress. One study, which focused on a sample of the general population with elevated levels of tension and anxiety, found that moderate aerobic training seemed to be associated with improvements in perceived ability to cope with stress and reductions in tension, anxiety, and depression.[50] The psychological improvements were found to be independent of fitness-changes, and it was thought that they might have emerged from factors such as a sense of achievement and positive feelings of self-control experienced by anxious people participating in training programmes.

It has also been suggested that hard cycling reduces tension: a group exercising for twenty minutes at 75-to-80 per cent intensity were found to have muscles twice as relaxed as a group exercising at 40 per cent intensity.[51] This decreased muscle tension presumably reflects a greater degree of relaxation and reduced stress.

Anecdotally, many people affirm that they 'feel good' during or for some time after exercise. Unfortunately, these subjective responses do not prove anything in the scientific sense. It may be that athletes are generally healthier than the majority of the population simply because they are the types who choose to become athletes.

However, there are some grounds for subscribing to the view that various forms of physical exercise contribute to mental well-being simply because of the positive enjoyment that people gain from them. It is for this reason that therapies such as running have been promoted in the US. Cycling as part of the daily routine is less likely to become compulsive, as can happen, albeit rarely, with other exercise patterns. It also confers a feeling of freedom and independence, and a sense of achievement derived from satisfying journey-needs entirely through one's own efforts. In this way, cycling could be viewed as a good way of starting the day in an alert and positive frame of mind and with a sense of achievement.

A study of attitudes to cycling recorded the great majority of respondents recalling the 'significant and pleasurable part' that it had played in their earlier lives and the 'exhilaration' they felt at the time.[52] It also established enjoyment, health, and independence as important reasons why cyclists choose to travel in this way in spite of the perceived danger of doing so, and recorded attractive symbolic connotations and associations of cycling with cleanliness, economy, freedom, youth, and 'doing your own thing'.

Whether anecdotal or experimental evidence is considered, it is becoming increasingly clear that exercise improves not only physical but also mental well-being. In these circumstances, it may be asked why more people do not do it: studies have shown that 70 per cent of participants drop out of exercise routines.[53] This may be explained first by situational factors, including accessibility—the further away a sports facility, the lower the participation rate[54] and the higher the drop-out rate[55]—as well as the number, intensity, and frequency of work-out sessions. Secondly, there are several participant reasons for drop-out, perhaps most importantly the one of low self-motivation, which tends to be explained as lack of time.

A recent report of the Royal College of Physicians has provided further evidence for the benefits of exercise to body and mind in healthy people and in those with medical conditions, including heart disease and asthma. The report concludes that: 'There is substantial evidence that regular aerobic exercise such as walking, jogging, dancing or swimming is beneficial to general physical and psychological health. Regular exercise appears to be particularly effective in prevention of coronary disease and osteoporosis and of some value in the management of obesity and diabetes.'[56]

Most of this chapter has been concerned with the general effects of exercise on health and fitness. The major themes that emerge from the evidence is that for exercise to be beneficial, it has to be regular, with an activity regimen maintained throughout life. To improve or maintain fitness, there is a threshold intensity level which must be exceeded, but this level is itself dependent on the initial fitness level. Thus, the kind of exercise which is likely to be ideal is one that can be conveniently undertaken on a day-to-day basis, with minimum interruption of the daily routine. It is obviously preferable for it to be inexpensive. Walking and cycling are examples of activities that meet these criteria for the majority of the population.

An increasing proportion of the population are becoming conscious of the benefits of exercise and are joining health-clubs and similar organizations—to which they may drive, pay a large fee, and then spend half an hour on a cycling machine! Given safe provision, cycling, as part of the daily routine, could represent an ideal, straightforward, and much more widely available means of maintaining fitness and gaining the other considerable health advantages set out in this chapter.

CHAPTER THREE

Current patterns of cycle ownership and use

It has been seen that substantial health and other societal benefits could be gained if more people were encouraged to adopt cycling as part of their daily routine. However, examination of statistics on cycle ownership and use shows that, whilst ownership is fairly high, the bicycle at present plays a very small part in daily routine and travel patterns.

Cycle ownership

The number of cycle-owning and multi-cycle-owning households is growing in spite of the largely deteriorating environment for cycling. The principal source of evidence on cycle ownership is that provided by manufacturers. Sales of bicycles have been rising fairly dramatically in recent years, from 0.6 million in 1969 to 1.5 million in 1985, and to 2.4 million in 1989; sales of 4 million have been forecast for 1993.[1] It is now thought that there are about 15 million cycles in use, not a significantly lower number than the 20 million cars on the road. The findings of the National Travel Surveys of 1975/6 and 1985/6 confirm this considerable increase in cycle ownership though they also reveal a far lower increase in cycle mileage. Table 3.1 shows that in the later survey for 1985/6, the findings of which are the most recently published, there had been an 80 per cent increase in the number of bicycles, a rise to more than a third of households owning at least one bicycle, but only a 16 per cent increase in cycle traffic.[2] However, in view of the rise in all road travel, the percentage of that undertaken by cycle has continued to fall.

A recent research survey found that in marked contrast to the car,

Table 3.1 Cycle ownership and cycle mileage, 1975/6, 1978/9, and 1985/6

	National Travel Surveys			% change
	1975/6	1978/9	1985/6	1975/6–1985/6
Number of cycles (millions)	7.32	9.47	13.14	+79
Cycle-owning households (%)	24	29	35	
Annual cycle traffic (billion km.)	3.99	4.03	4.44	+16
Cycle travel as proportion of all mechanical road travel (%)	1.8	1.7	1.6	

Sources: J. M. Morgan, 'How many cyclists and how many bicycles are there in Great Britain?', unpublished working paper WP(TP) 36 (Transport and Road Research Laboratory, Crowthorne, 1987); Department of Transport, *Transport Statistics Great Britain* (HMSO, London, 1990).

where 94 per cent are used every day,[3] only one in three bicycles are used in a typical week.[4] In fact, it has been calculated that nearly four million bicycles are used at least once a week, just under a third of them for commuting to work. More recently, a survey undertaken in a sample of schools around the country ranging from an inner London suburb to a rural area of Oxfordshire recorded cycle-ownership levels of 90 per cent among the junior and 76 per cent among the senior schoolchildren.[5]

Cycle use

Until the National Travel Surveys first covered all travel, including journeys of under one mile, in 1972/3, little evidence was available on patterns of cycling, other than estimates of mileage based on the number of vehicles crossing road cordons. Comparison of the record of cycle travel from these counts with the findings of the National Travel Surveys shows that cycling plays a significantly lower part in the overall pattern of travel than it used to. In 1949, 34 per cent of travel mileage by mechanical modes was made by bicycle, the majority on commuter journeys. By 1969 only 2 per cent were made by bicycle, and now only 1 per cent. Between the surveys of 1975/6 and

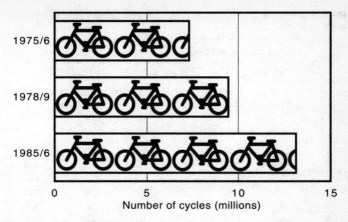

Figure 3.1 Cycle ownership
The National Travel Surveys have shown a considerable increase in cycle ownership, with the most recently published figures revealing an 80% increase over the ten year period 1975/6 to 1985/6. However, there has been a far lower increase in cycle mileage with cycling representing only a very small proportion of all road travel. *Sources*: as for Table 3.1.

1985/6, both mileage per cycle and cycle trips per week were almost halved.[6] Although about a third of cycle journeys are made over distances of one-and-a-half kilometres, their average length is currently just under three kilometres, that is about a ten-minute ride.

Table 3.2 shows the proportion of all journeys that are made by cycle and the number of journeys made by cycle per week by each age-band and by gender, and the changes in these two measures that occurred during the ten-year period. It can be seen that cycling has a very low share in the patterns of travel of each population group. The frequency of average cycle journeys per week has hardly changed but, because the total number of journeys has increased markedly, the proportion made by cycle has fallen by over a quarter.

Closer examination of the figures in the Table shows that the only age/gender group which makes more than a very small proportion of its journeys by bicycle are young male teenagers between the ages of 11 and 15, who make about one in seven of their journeys in this way. The findings of significant change in the ten-year period in the amount of cycling among such groups as young girls and women pen-

Table 3.2 Patterns of cycle travel according to age and gender, 1975/6 and 1985/6

| | Cycle journeys per week | | | | | |
| | 1975/6 | | 1985/6 | | 1975/6–1985/6 | |
Age in years	% of all journeys	Number	% of all journeys	Number	% change of all journeys	Number
Male						
5–10	3.5	0.44	2.1	0.36	−40	−18
11–15	14.8	2.22	13.4	2.74	−9	+24
16–20	5.3	0.86	5.9	1.31	+11	+53
21–29	2.2	0.40	2.6	0.61	+18	+53
30–59	3.1	0.56	2.1	0.51	−32	−10
60–64	4.7	0.74	2.1	0.41	−55	−45
65 and over	4.3	0.50	2.2	0.35	−49	−30
All	4.4	0.70	3.2	0.68	−27	−3
Female						
5–10	1.8	0.12	1.3	0.23	−28	+88
11–15	4.7	0.75	3.8	0.81	−19	+9
16–20	1.8	0.29	1.8	0.42	0	+46
21–29	1.0	0.17	1.3	0.30	+30	+78
30–59	2.7	0.41	1.5	0.32	−44	−22
60–64	1.8	0.22	1.3	0.20	−28	−8
65 and over	0.5	0.04	0.5	0.06	0	+38
All	2.1	0.31	1.5	0.29	−28	−6
TOTAL	3.3	0.49	2.4	0.48	−27	−3

Source: Department of Transport, *Transport Statistics Great Britain* (HMSO, London, 1990).

sioners needs to be treated with caution, as the calculations are based on very low frequencies of weekly journeys on bicycles.

Table 3.3 records the role of cycling, walking, and the car for each of the principal types of journey that people made in the two surveys. It can be seen that, in both surveys, cycles are mainly used for commuting, though even in this case, in 1985/6, cycle travel only accounted for 4.6 per cent of journeys to and from work. The other main use of cycles is for educational journeys, including school and adult education. They are rarely used on other journeys, including those for leisure for which they could be considered to be particularly appropriate, though it should be noted that a report forming part of the General Household Survey shows a marked increase in cycle travel for this purpose.[7]

Comparison of patterns of travel during the ten-year period reveal a general decline in the use of bicycles for all journey purposes other than the small increase in the few made in the course of work. Indeed, as cycle ownership has grown so significantly between the dates of the two surveys, it can be calculated that the average distance travelled per cycle has been halved.

Table 3.3 Method of travel according to journey purpose, 1975/6 and 1985/6

Journey purpose	% of 1975/6 journeys			% of 1985/6 journeys		
	Cycle	Walk	Car	Cycle	Walk	Car
Work	5.6	19.1	50.2	4.6	17.8	54.2
Course of work	1.7	11.6	77.0	2.1	11.0	65.8
Education	4.0	59.8	12.8	3.6	55.6	18.0
Shopping	2.3	45.7	34.2	1.6	46.9	37.8
Personal business	3.8	37.1	44.8	1.7	35.2	50.2
Social	2.4	25.9	56.5	2.4	27.9	57.1
Escorting	0.8	29.0	66.5	0.4	30.8	63.5
Other leisure	2.4	41.5	43.4	1.5	46.0	42.9
TOTAL	3.3	34.6	44.7	2.4	35.4	47.6

Note: Proportions do not total 100 as they exclude journeys by other means, particularly public transport.
Source: Department of Transport, *Transport Statistics Great Britain* (HMSO, London, 1990).

Deterrents to cycling

It is quite clear that the low use of bicycles set against the high level of ownership outlined in Chapter 3 is explained by concerns about the consequences of actually using them as a form of transport rather than as an item of recreational equipment. Examination of the variations in levels of cycling in different areas[1] and responses to attitudinal surveys about cycling[2] indicate that the principal factors deterring people from cycling are the risk of accident, exposure to traffic fumes, dislike of the physical effort required in cycling—particularly in hilly areas—inclement weather, cycle theft, social attitudes, and the wider availability of cars and public transport. This chapter is concerned with all but the first two of these factors, which are dealt with in depth in the following two chapters.

Effort

The effort involved in cycling clearly correlates with distance travelled, so that the longer the journey that has to be made the less likely it is that the cycle will be seen to be an appropriate mode of travel. Table 4.1 shows the distribution by distance-band of cycle journeys. Two-thirds of these journeys are currently less than 3.2 kilometres long—a ten- to twelve-minute ride—and nearly all of them are less than 8 kilometres long—a twenty- to thirty-minute ride. From this, it can be inferred that for the great majority of cyclists, a ride of 8 kilometres generally represents an upper limit to the distance they are prepared to ride.

Analysis of data from the 1981 Census shows the proportion of people cycling to work in England and Wales ranging from 13 per cent in

Table 4.1 Proportion of journeys by cycle and by all travel methods according to distance-band (%)

	Distance band (km.)		
	up to 3.2	3.2 to 8.0	8.0 and over
Cycle	69.2	24.8	6.0
All travel methods	51.6	24.1	24.3

Source: Department of Transport, *National Travel Survey: 1985/86 Report—Part 1: An Analysis of Personal Travel* (HMSO, London, 1988).

Cambridgeshire to less than 1 per cent in Glamorgan.[3] National Travel Survey findings also show what might be intuitively felt, namely that cycle ownership and use are more common in the flatter rather than the hilly regions of the country. For instance, 50 per cent of households in East Anglia are cycle-owning in contrast to 33 per cent in Wales.[4] Similar results were found in surveys in West Germany, which recorded the incidence of cycling to be 50 per cent above average in flat terrain and 20 per cent below average in mountain areas.[5]

It should be noted, however, that advances in cycle technology over the last few decades, particularly with regard to gears and the weight of bicycles, have reduced considerably the effort involved in cycling up hills. In addition, well-designed panniers and highly efficient trailers now make it possible to carry quite heavy loads without difficulty.

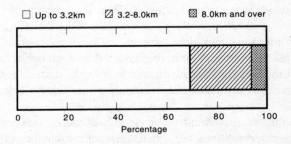

Figure 4.1 Proportion of journeys by cycle according to distance
Quite clearly most journeys made by cycle are over distances of less than 8 km. Such figures indicate that for journeys of up to 8 km cycling is an appropriate means of travel. *Source*: Department of Transport, *National Travel Survey: 1985/86 Report—Part 1: An Analysis of Personal Travel* (HMSO, London, 1988).

Climate

A further reason cited by people for not cycling is a dislike of doing so in adverse weather conditions: rainfall, high temperatures in the summer, and low temperatures sometimes associated with snow and ice on the roads in the winter, may all act as deterrents. Nevertheless, data from the Meteorological Office show that rainfall is fairly infrequent,[6] with the average number of rainy days (defined by the amount and duration of at least two hours between 7 a.m. and 5 p.m., but excluding those hours with less than 0.2 mm of rain) even in Glasgow, which has about 50 per cent more rainfall than London, being only fifty-two a year. Indeed, the incidence of rain on a typical cycle journey is very low: on average, the likelihood of rainfall during a ten-minute period in south-east England is only about one in a hundred,[7] and of course lower still if some flexibility can be built into the time of departure to avoid it. However, even if it only rains for a few minutes during a cycle journey the overall effect can be rather unpleasant.

Records of the extent of snow in Britain in the most recent thirty-year period for which figures are available, show that, even in north England and south Scotland, snow fell on average on only eight or nine days and lay for only twelve to thirteen days each year. The figures for Wales and the Midlands were about half of this, and were lower still for southern England.[8]

As far as low temperatures are concerned, the data show that, even in January and February, the coldest months of the year, the average twenty-four-hour minimum temperature is several degrees centigrade above freezing point in England, and only just below freezing point in some parts of Scotland, and in any case, daytime temperatures, though not published, are certainly several degrees higher than this.

A further factor to consider is that feelings of cold are exaggerated in wet or windy conditions. The, albeit fairly rare, combination of low air temperature and high wind speed in dry and wet conditions intensifies discomfort. Some indication of the dramatic effect of wind chill, and the even more dramatic effect of moisture, is apparent from the fact that if the air temperature is 5 degrees centigrade—a cold but not freezing day—freewheeling downhill at 50 kph can induce the feeling of a temperature of minus-11 degrees centigrade. But if it is raining, even a mild 15 degrees centigrade would induce a feeling of a temperature below freezing.[9]

However, most regular cyclists consider that low temperatures rarely pose a problem as, for winter cycling, the quality of protective wind- and rainproof clothing and gloves, consisting of several layers of finely woven material, has minimized the problem. Although low temperatures may not pose an insurmountable problem to cyclists' comfort, they can create significant hazards for them. Temperatures may rarely drop below freezing during the day, but ice which has formed overnight will nevertheless create a hazard for those cycling in the morning, such as commuters.

The discomfort of cycling in hot weather, due to overheating and excess perspiration, is relatively rare owing to Britain's temperate summers and the fact that commuting-times do not coincide with the hottest part of the day, generally between 2 p.m. and 3 p.m. In fact, there is more cycling in the summer months than in the winter months, principally because cycles are used more for recreational purposes at that time of year, rather than because they are used less for commuting in winter months.

Cycle theft

A further deterrent to cycling is the fear of theft. The most recent figures on this show that concern on this aspect of cycling is justifiable: 387,000 cycles were reported stolen in England and Wales in 1989,[10] and this represents a significant increase on the number stolen ten years previously.[11] Two further factors reinforce this concern. First, well under half this number are reported to the police.[12] Secondly, only about one in ten of the reported thefts are recovered and returned to their owner.[13] Despite publicity, police campaigns, much-improved locks, and post-coding which makes it much more likely that, once found, bicycles are returned to their owners, cycle theft continues to rise and discourages people from cycling where there is insufficient security at their destination. It should be mentioned within this context that cycle insurance, enabling cycles to be replaced if stolen, is now widely available.

Work environment

People may be deterred from commuting to work by bicycle due to in-adequate facilities at their work-place. Basic resources are needed, such as secure bicycle-storage facilities (preferably with racks), showers, and changing rooms as well as storage space for work-clothes and cycle accessories such as helmets, cycle pumps, and lights. A six-point charter for employers has recently been produced by the London Cycling Campaign giving guidance on the provision of such work-place facilities for cyclists.[14] These amenities would not have large cost implications for the employer, and as well as improving the lot of the working cyclist, they could prove beneficial to the company through improved health and fitness of the work-force. Due to the health benefits of cycling both for the individual and for the wider community, Health Authorities could take an important lead in providing such facilities.

Attitudes

Transport behaviour is based on perceived needs and subjective beliefs of how travel needs can be satisfied. Although beliefs and perceived needs can be more or less accurate, they are also subject to earlier experiences, personal values, the adequacy of information, and deeply rooted habits, and these can influence whether people even consider using bicycles to get around. Besides these individual psychological factors, social factors play a crucial role. The direct social environment, such as family, friends, and colleagues, and the larger social context mediate the information people receive and set norms determining which beliefs and behaviour are proper.[15]

One of the major and obvious deterrents to cycling in the last few decades has been the growing availability of cars and, concomitantly, public attitudes to cyclists as 'second class' road-users compared with motorists. However, this now seems to be changing as the inability to sustain traffic-growth is becoming better recognized and its adverse impacts better understood. It may be that this process will accelerate as the advantages of cycling as a means of maintaining fitness become more widely appreciated at the same time as widespread public provision for it is made. This could alter perception of what is reasonable and normal travel behaviour. Thus, attitudes to cycling, while to some extent formed personally, are also in fact socially conditioned. Cultures in which the bicycle is socially acceptable as a form of transport, as in Denmark and the Netherlands, have much higher proportions of cyclists than those in which it is not.

From a psychological rather than a social viewpoint, attitudes are also rooted in experiences of childhood. The ambition of most children is to own a bicycle, and for a large majority this is fulfilled. In a survey of schoolchildren in different areas of England, 90 per cent of the juniors and 76 per cent of the seniors reported that they were cycle owners.[16] It might therefore be supposed that the children would become accustomed to using a bicycle as transport and that this view of the uses of a bicycle would pervade their later life. However, the survey found that three-quarters of the junior-school owners and a quarter of the senior-school owners were not allowed by their parents to use their cycles on the roads. It is clear that these bicycles were used mainly as playthings rather than as transport. Where the seniors might have been expected to use them as transport, for instance on their journey to school, very few of them did so, even though about three in five of the cycle owners had journeys of less than two kilometres, which is an easy distance to cycle given safe conditions.[17]

The parental restrictions are perhaps less surprising when one considers that children use adults as models, and that although the majority of children own bicycles, the proportion of adults who cycle is very small. For this reason, most children have little or no experience of their parents using cycles for transport. They are more likely to have been taken with their bicycles, with their parents walking along with them, to a place where they could use them safely.

That attitudes to bicycles and cycling appear to stem from a perspective of bicycles being principally for children was confirmed in a study carried out to identify the main factors influencing the amount of cycling in order to determine future demand.[18] It was found that adults associate cycling with a pleasurable part of their childhood. It was a way of developing practical skills and techniques and achieving status, as well as a means of transport enabling them to be less dependent on parents. It was not a family activity. There was a stigma attached to not owning a bicycle or not being able to ride one at the age of 7 or 8. Most of the adult respondents had both cycled and enjoyed it, but had then tended to outgrow it during their adolescent years when it was seen to be 'childish', fitting neither the desired 'macho' image of the boys nor the sophisticated one desired by the girls.[19]

Slightly older respondents became more influenced by practical considerations. Many factors in life-style were not conducive to the use of bicycles, and status demanded a car rather than a bike. For somewhat older respondents, especially those with families, the car or public transport were seen to be more suitable, for instance, for shopping or family-travel needs. It simply did not occur to many of them that the bicycle was a serious form of transport that they could use. To a certain extent the use of specially designed child-seats on bicycles can meet the requirement for family travel. Parents need be no more worried about taking their children by bicycle than by other means of transport, provided proper precautions regarding the type of child-seat used, the condition of the bicycle, protective clothing, and choice of route are taken. Detailed guidance on the safe means of carrying children on bicycles is available from the Royal Society for the Prevention of Accidents.

To some extent, the non-cyclists' image of cyclists reflected these attitudes; cyclists were considered to be children, students, cycling and keep-fit enthusiasts, and those who were not very well-off. On the other hand, the cyclists' image of cyclists was as a minority group. Some of them felt a sense of achievement in travelling under their own energy and being in total control. Some considered it stylish to be cyclists and suspected that, even though non-cyclists might regard them as eccentric, they were in some ways admired. Cyclists were found in all age-groups, some cycling because they could not afford motorized transport, some out of choice, and some for recreation. Others had started out of necessity and, having become accustomed to it, had continued to do so.

Attitudes varied by gender, women seeming to be more timid about cycling, stressing the effort and discomfort. The 'sporty' image was seen to be more appropriate to men, who regarded the bicycle as a functional object. Men, especially younger ones, were more likely to be concerned about the model of bicycle and did more cycle maintenance. The benefits of cycling were seen in terms of saving money, exercise, and convenience. The enjoyment of being out in the open, rather than 'boxed-in', was an added benefit for some, offering the opportunity to notice surroundings and providing a feeling of freedom. A few also mentioned environmental benefits—less noise and danger—through cycling rather than driving .

Three main practical disadvantages to cycling were established. First, it was seen to entail some physical effort and inconvenience on longer journeys or when things had to be carried. Secondly, it could be unpleasant in certain road and weather conditions. Thirdly, vulnerability from other traffic was quoted, with people expressing fear as a reason for not cycling. Less mention was made of the health-hazards of exhaust fumes, the problem of cycle theft, and the mechanical knowledge required. Some thought that cycling was not socially acceptable.

The report by Finch and Morgan concluded:

Taking into account all the attitudes expressed, it seems that one of the most important requirements in promoting cycling among adults would be to encourage them to consider it at all as a possible means of transport for use in adult life . . . It is clear that the low social status accorded to cycling by many adult respondents is a major dissuasive factor, at least as powerful as their expressed concerns about danger from other traffic and the physical discomforts involved . . . only by creating for it a fashionable image could it begin to be encouraged.[20]

At the time that the findings of this survey were published in 1985, it is clear that the question of whether cycling was generally considered in the context of transport at all was not addressed. The bicycle was simply not a part of the adult British culture. It seems likely that younger respondents were far more accustomed to travel by car, with its attendant comforts, and thus more likely to regard cycling as involving unacceptable effort and exposure to bad weather. Even those who did not drive were mostly expecting to do so at some stage and expressed no intention of buying a bicycle.

Alternatives often only become apparent when they are seen to be a realistic and appropriate option. The foremost instance of changing attitudes to the bicycle which has developed in recent years is in the commercial sector. Firms wanting messages delivered quickly in

41

cities are now using cycle couriers: bicycles have been found to be faster and more reliable than motorized means of transport. During the London rail stoppages of 1989, a significant number of commuters appeared in the streets on bicycles. They were then seen to be an appropriate and acceptable means of travel. Some continued to cycle even after the initial reason for doing so had gone away, as their experience had in some ways modified their attitude. It may be that many more, if provided with good cycling facilities, would have become regular cyclists.

In recent years there has been a significant growth in environmental awareness, particularly with regard to the disadvantages of the car as a common form of transport. In countries such as Denmark and Germany, where this awareness has a longer history, cycling has increasingly been encouraged and is no longer viewed as the activity of a fringe group. The growth of lobbies formed to promote the interests of cyclists, and the positive response of central and local government to the strength of their arguments, may have helped to change public attitudes to cycling, particularly in conjunction with growing consciousness of its health and environmental benefits.

Another set of attitudes which has been progressively changing relates to appearance. A track-suit and trainers, which are in many ways ideal cycle-wear, are no longer regarded as solely the dress of the athlete, and it is interesting to note the recent popularity of cycle-wear as 'high-fashion' for the non-cyclist. It is possible to look attractive and have some sex-appeal in these kinds of clothes, and this is how they are marketed. In many jobs, too, the compulsion to dress formally for daily wear, for instance for men to dress in a suit and tie, appears to be less strongly felt than it used to be. It is now acceptable for women to wear trousers, and this again means that the deterrence to cycling of not being formally dressed is less than it once was.

The advent of the Mountain Bike (ATB, All Terrain Bike) in recent years has seen cycling being marketed in ways designed to create a fashionable, sporty, and in some cases macho image. Sales of Mountain Bikes would suggest that this approach has been successful. However, it is important when fashionable images are being created that safety is given equal importance, and dangerous cycling is not encouraged by the advertisers.

Enjoyment, health, cheapness, and independence—in that order—were most frequently cited as advantages of cycling. Not surprisingly, members of cycling clubs stressed enjoyment while other cyclists stressed the more functional aspects of cycling. Some of the reasons for cycling were age-dependent: younger cyclists between the ages of 20 and 29 cycled for the sake of cheapness, but those in their forties rated the health-benefits much more highly.[21]

A comparison of attitudes to cycling in the EC member states shows that, in Denmark, the Netherlands, and Italy, bicycles are regarded as part and parcel of everyday transport,[22] and cyclists in the Netherlands, Denmark, and in (West) Germany feel respected. Cyclists in this country, on the other hand, feel less respected than any of their counterparts in other member states.

Perhaps the importance of culture and attitudes to cycling is best illustrated by reference to changes that have occurred in the last few decades in the Netherlands. In the 1950s the bicycle there was regarded as a mode of transport for the poor, but the high level of provision for it—the densest cycle network in the world—has led to its status growing steadily and to it having almost wholly positive images in terms of aiding fitness and being environmentally friendly as well as convenient and fast.[23] Weather is rarely mentioned as a problem, and there is little concern regarding traffic safety because the bicycle is regularly used and integrated into daily traffic and society in general. The only real concern is with theft, which is very common.

People's awareness of cyclists would clearly be heightened by getting them on to bicycles: people are simply not accustomed to cycling, and this represents a major stumbling-block. If they could be persuaded to cycle, and thereby derive the benefits of doing so, at the least this could improve their tolerance of cyclists as road-users with rights, and could encourage them to recognize that cycling is a realistic alternative to motorized transport.

CHAPTER FIVE

Danger on the road

Any analysis of the public-health aspects of cycling, and the proposition that cycling should be promoted in order to derive the benefits, especially to health, of doing so, must be made in the context of the risks of being involved in a road accident. Cycle accidents are not uncommon; one survey found that nearly one in three cyclists had been involved in some kind of accident.[1] Indeed, the primary reason that people give for not cycling is the fear of this happening. This chapter examines the pattern of road accidents to reveal how far that fear is justified, who is involved in road accidents, and when and where they occur.

Growth in the volume and speed of traffic in the last few decades has certainly made the cycling environment increasingly unsafe. However, that is not necessarily revealed in the incidence of accidents. The very obvious increase in threat posed by traffic growth has discouraged some people from cycling. Those who continue to cycle may compensate for the unsafe environment by exercising ever-greater care rather than perhaps cycling in a more relaxed frame of mind.

Road-accident data

Over recent years the number of road-users killed and injured has declined, despite the greater numbers on the roads, so that the risk for each individual road-user is lower. Indeed, the number of people killed on the roads in Britain reached a peak of 7,985 in 1966, since which time the absolute numbers of deaths, injuries, and crashes have gradually but steadily declined. Of those road-users who are killed in Britain, the largest proportion (43 per cent) are the occupants of cars, followed by pedestrians (33 per cent), motor-cyclists (14 per cent) and pedal cyclists (5.5 per cent).[2] Whilst cyclists are not the greatest proportion of all road-traffic accidents, the smaller number of cyclists on the road means that cycling has a comparatively higher risk of death than other modes of transport.

There are a variety of ways of recording the risk of cycling compared with that of travelling by other modes. They can be measured according to the casualty-rate per capita, per hour of exposure, or per journey. One of the most direct ways, however, is to compare them according to the number per vehicle-kilometre travelled.

The main source of road-accident data in Britain is the information collected by the police in their reports of accidents involving death or injury. These are reported on the Department of Transport forms—'Stats 19',[3] although it should be noted that a considerable number of cycling accidents are not reported to the police. Department of Transport figures for cycling accidents are therefore likely to underestimate the true level of cycling incidents and as such are somewhat unreliable. Table 5.1 shows how the reported number of cycle deaths and injuries has changed over the last ten years and how the proportion of fatalities has varied.

It can be seen that, with the exception of the most recent figures, both cycle fatalities and injuries of all severities per kilometre travelled have fluctuated during the decade, but that the fatality-rate as a proportion of all severities has tended to fall. This could either reflect

Table 5.1 Cycle fatalities and injuries per 100 million vehicle km., 1979–1989

	Rate per 100 million vehicle km.										
	1979	1980	1981	1982	1983	1984	1985	1986	1987	1988	1989
Fatalities	7.0	5.9	5.7	4.6	5.1	5.4	4.7	5.0	4.9	4.3	5.7
Injuries of all severity	517	487	465	440	480	485	446	479	457	494	552
Fatalities as % of injuries of all severity	1.35	1.21	1.22	1.05	1.06	1.11	1.05	1.04	1.07	0.87	1.03

Source: Department of Transport, *Road Accidents Great Britain: The Casualty Report* (HMSO, London, 1990); also earlier annual volumes.

Table 5.2 Casualty-rates per 100 million km. travelled as cyclist and car driver, 1969, 1979, and 1989

	per 100 million km. travelled		
	1969	1979	1989
Fatality rate			
(a) Cycle	8.0	7.0	5.7
(b) Car driver	0.9	0.7	0.5
Ratio (a) to (b)	8.9	10.0	11.4
Serious-injury rate			
(a) Cycle	110.0	108.0	93.3
(b) Car driver	12.0	9.3	4.5
Ratio (a) to (b)	9.2	11.6	20.7

Source: Department of Transport, *Road Accidents Great Britain: The Casualty Report* (HMSO, London,1990); also earlier annual volumes.

an increase in medical skills, so that those severely injured are nowadays more likely to survive, or it could reflect an increase in the reporting of accidents involving cyclists.

Casualty-rates per kilometre travelled by different travel methods can also be compared in order to show the wide range in the level of risk, although it should be noted that comparing accident-rates per 100 million kilometres between different road-users can be misleading. The risk to cyclists may be exaggerated as they are actually exposed to the danger for much longer periods of time than a car-driver in travelling the same distance. This problem is illustrative of the inherent difficulties of using comparative safety statistics for different road-users. Such difficulties have been addressed by the Department of Transport in the most recent transport statistics.[4] In this report comparative accident-rates for passengers by mode of transport are examined. The 'traditional' approach to risk analysis shows cyclists are 11.5 times more likely to be killed, per passenger-kilometre, than car users. However, it is shown that this ratio falls to 2.4 if 'trips' are used as the comparative basis, or to 5.2 if time-exposure is used. The use of relative-risk statistics have an important bearing on public attitudes and the acceptability of cycling as a viable means of transport; as such their limitations must be understood. A useful guide to the problems of measuring road safety through statistical information is presented in a recent book edited by R. D. Tolley.[5]

Table 5.2 suggests that, in current traffic conditions which rarely provide for cycle routes away from motor vehicles, the fatality rate per kilometre travelled by cycle is about 11 times higher than that for a car driver, and that the serious-injury rate is over 20 times higher. Whilst it is apparent from the Table that the casualty-rates for cycling over the last twenty years have been falling, cyclists have benefited least as it can be seen that the gap between the safety of cyclists and of car drivers has widened substantially during the period. For instance, whereas the serious-injury rate for cyclists was nine times as high as that for car drivers in 1969, it had more than doubled by 1989. It is important to note that approximately three-quarters of all cycle fatalities and serious injuries occur as a result of a collision with a car.

As traffic counts, including those covering cyclists, are unable to include a record of the age of the road-user, there are no statistics on the cycle casualty-rate per kilometre travelled for each age-group. However, figures are recorded on the rate per 100,000 of the population. Table 5.3, based on these figures, shows a much higher fatality and serious-injury rate among child cyclists compared with adult cyclists. When it is borne in mind that the distance cycled by children and adults is not dissimilar—the National Travel Survey records the average weekly cycle-travel of children as 1.3 kilometres and that of adults of working age at 1.6 kilometres[6]—it is apparent that children are many times more at risk of injury than are adults. Those age-groups with the greatest cycling casualty-rates are therefore those for which motor vehicles are not a possible means of independent travel; the legal driving age in the UK being 17. This fact should be borne in mind when attempting to compare the relative risks of motorized transport and cycling, as for those suffering the highest cycling casualty-rate no such direct comparison can be made.

Table 5.3 Cycle casualty-rate per 100,000 population by age-group

Accident severity	per 100,000 population								
	5–9	10–14	15–19	20–9	30–9	40–9	50–9	60–9	70+
Fatal	0.3	1.5	1.0	0.4	0.3	0.4	0.4	0.6	0.8
Fatal and serious	11.0	29.0	25.0	11.0	7.0	6.0	6.0	5.0	4.0

Source: Department of Transport, *Road Accidents Great Britain: The Casualty Report* (HMSO, London, 1990); also earlier annual volumes.

In fact, the cycle casualty-rate peaks in the age-group 12 to 15 for both males and females, reflecting the higher levels of cycling on the road by this age-group, and perhaps their more daredevil behaviour.[7]

Although it is unlikely to invalidate the general thrust of the findings noted above, care must be exercised in comparing road-accident statistics for several reasons. First, there is a wide level of under-reporting of injuries; secondly, there are varying definitions of injury severity; and thirdly, revisions have been made to the published figures on annual cycle mileage as traffic counts on main-road cordons over the years have been found to have missed a large amount of cycling, a relatively high proportion of which is made on minor roads. Indeed, the problem of identifying where cycle accidents take place is also not straightforward for these reasons.

Under-reporting of accidents

The principal problem is the extent to which the under-reporting of accidents varies with different travel methods, situations, and severities of injury. There is much evidence that people do not always report cycle accidents. Several studies have compared the number reported by the police with the number treated in hospital for injuries. The findings of these studies were fairly similar.[8] A more recent study showed that 74 per cent of the 'slight reportable accidents' and 61 per cent of the 'serious reportable accidents' go unreported. The report concluded that the total number of pedal-cycle accidents per year could be around 87,000 rather than the 26,000 reported in the national statistics.[9]

The Department of Trade and Industry Consumer Safety Unit collects data on home and leisure accidents, including cycling. This Leisure Accidents Surveillance System (LASS) involves twenty-two hospitals and monitors patients arriving at Accident and Emergency departments, identifying cycling injuries among other accidents arising from leisure pursuits. It therefore records those cycling accidents that would otherwise go unreported.

Table 5.4, although containing the results of only one study, provides evidence that very few cyclists treated in hospital who sustain serious or slight injuries are recorded on police statistics forms, and therefore in the Department of Transport's figures on road accidents.

Table 5.4 Under-reporting by injury severity of pedal-cycle casualties in potentially reportable pedal-cycle accidents

Severity	Police-reported	Not police-reported	Total	Level of under-reporting (%)
	No. (%)	No. (%)	No. (%)	
Slight	105 (48)	293 (63)	398 (58)	74
Serious	112 (51)	173 (37)	285 (42)	61
Fatal	2 (1)	0 (0)	2 (<1)	0
TOTAL	219 (100)	466 (100)	685 (100)	68

Source: P. J. Mills, *Pedal Cycle Accidents—A Hospital Based Study*, TRRL 220 (Transport and Road Research Laboratory, Crowthorne, 1989).

With such marked discrepancies in the data, it is necessary to use several sources to get a clearer picture than can be provided by road-accident statistics. First, however, it should be noted that there is no under-reporting of fatalities, and some interesting conclusions can be drawn from these. Most journeys by cycle are made in urban areas. From 1986 to 1989 inclusive, 1,072 cyclists were recorded as being killed, and 105,613 were injured. Of these, 60 per cent of those killed and 90 per cent of those injured occurred in built-up areas (defined as areas with a speed-limit of 40 mph or less). The figures suggest that the reason for the much higher ratio of fatalities to injury is less a matter of traffic density, road layout, or type of manœuvre than it is of the speed that vehicles are travelling when they collide with cyclists. These findings are not unique to Britain. In Sweden and the Netherlands, the ratio of fatalities to injuries of all severities is about five times higher in non-urban areas, where speed is not controlled, than in urban areas.[10] This provides further justification for wide programmes of traffic-calming measures in order to ensure that traffic moves more slowly, thereby allowing more time for drivers to take evasive action.

Location of cycle accidents

Table 5.5 shows that young children under 10 have most of their accidents on unclassified roads,[11] but adults have accidents on A Class roads—not surprisingly, in view of the restrictions on where children

Table 5.5 Pedal-cyclist casualties according to age-group and class of road

Age-group	Class of road					
	C and unclassified		A, A (M), and M*		B	
	No.	(%)	No.	(%)	No.	(%)
0–9	2,173	(80)	361	(13)	180	(7)
10–14	4,560	(57)	2,409	(30)	991	(12)
15+	7,458	(38)	9,697	(50)	2,378	(12)
Unspecified	142	(38)	190	(51)	37	(10)
TOTAL	14,333	(47)	12,657	(41)	3,586	(12)

Note: *21 casualties were recorded on A (M) or M roads.
Source: C. S. Downing, *Pedal Cycling Accidents in Great Britain, Ways to Safer Cycling: Conference Proceedings* (Department of Transport, London, 1985).

can ride and the way in which they are allowed, generally by their parents, to use their bicycles.

Published figures suggest that about 70 per cent of all cycling accidents in Britain take place at or close to junctions.[12] However, two other studies, based on hospital records, have found much lower proportions occurring at these locations.[13] Table 5.6 shows that most junction cycling accidents occur at T-junctions, probably because this is the most common type of junction.

Clusters of cycling accidents, that is three or more over a three-year period at a specific junction, appear to be rare and occur mainly at roundabouts.[14] Although there are far less roundabouts than T-junctions, they pose a higher risk of accident for cyclists. A study at four-arm roundabouts showed that cyclists face ten to fifteen times the risk of being involved in an accident than do car occupants for every journey through the roundabouts.[15] Most of this type of accident occurs as a result of circulating cyclists being hit by vehicles entering roundabouts.[16] A recent review of literature concluded that cyclist accident-rates at roundabouts are up to fifteen times those for cars and two to three times those for cyclists at traffic signals. The report recommended that a substantial programme of remedial measures to improve safety at roundabouts was justified by the data on accidents.[17]

The most common cause of cycling accidents at T-junctions is when a vehicle emerging from a minor road is in collision with a cyclist on the major road.[18] The second most common cause (12 per

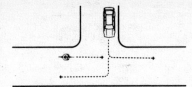

1. Motorist emerging into path of cyclist going straight ahead

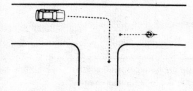

2. Motorist turning right into side road, cyclist going straight ahead

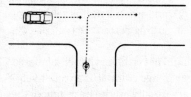

3. Cyclist emerging from side road, motorist going straight ahead

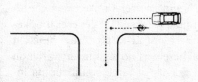

4. Motorist turning left into side road, cyclist going straight ahead

Figure 5.1 Common types of cycling accidents at T- junctions

Published figures indicate that 70 per cent of all cycling accidents in Britain take place at or close to junctions. Accidents at T- junctions are particularly common and such junctions can be hazardous to cyclists for a number of different reasons. Most commonly a vehicle emerging from a minor road collides with a cyclist on the major road. Reproduced from the 'Cycleway Tutor's Guide' with the kind permission of RoSPA.

Table 5.6 Pedal-cyclist casualties in relation to junction detail

Junction detail	1983, Stats 19 data	
	No.	(%)
T or staggered junction	12,705	(42)
Not at or within 20 metres of junction	8,596	(28)
Crossroads	3,430	(11)
Roundabout	1,998	(7)
Using private drive or entrance	1,909	(6)
Other junction	595	(2)
Y-junction	522	(2)
Multiple junction	374	(1)
Mini-roundabout	240	(1)
Slip-road	207	(1)

Source: Department of Transport, *Road Accidents Great Britain: The Casualty Report* (HMSO, London, 1990), also earlier annual volumes.

cent), is when a motor vehicle approaching on a major road and turning right is in collision with an oncoming cyclist. Other locations of accidents include when cyclists emerge from a minor road at a T-junction and are in collision with a motor vehicle travelling from offside on a major road (10 per cent), and when a motor vehicle approaching on a major road turns left, cutting across the path of a cyclist (6 per cent) (See Figure 5.1).

In examining such statistics it should nevertheless be remembered that the bicycle has a relatively small image compared to other vehicles on the road, and that cyclists are usually on the near-side of the road so that they are on the periphery of a driver's vision or obscured by roadside objects or other vehicles. Even if the cyclist has taken measures to increase his conspicuity the motorist may still have no time to take avoiding action due to such poor visibility.

A survey of nearly 9,000 people found a correlation between the location of accidents and cyclists' annual mileage.[19] In general, the likelihood of being involved in an accident at a 'give-way' junction decreased with annual mileage. There was no significant variation with small roundabouts, but accidents at large roundabouts increased with annual mileage. No clear pattern emerged with cycle accidents at slip-roads or traffic signals. These junctions appeared to create problems for all groups of cyclists, no matter what their annual mileage. Thus, it was found that experience has some bearing on where accidents take place—as has been seen, so does age. The contribution of road conditions to cycle accidents where another vehicle is involved is also unclear owing to an insufficiency of data. For instance, a cyclist may swerve to avoid a pot-hole and collide with a car, but the police report on this is unlikely to refer to the pot-hole.

Factors contributing to accidents

Although alcohol's contribution to road-traffic accidents is commonly associated with motorists, it should be noted that 12 per cent of cyclist fatalities have blood-alcohol concentrations exceeding the legal limit of 80 mg/100 ml.[20] Alcohol consumption by cyclists themselves, as well as by motorists, is therefore a contributory factor to cycling accidents and fatalities.

When cycle accidents not involving motor vehicles are considered, other factors come into play. Table 5.7, though based on a small sample, suggests that control skills, or lack of them, and use of cycles for play have some influence on the frequency of minor accidents.

Table 5.7 Main contributory factors in pedal-cycling accidents involving no motor vehicle

Main contributory factor	Cyclist casualties	
	No.	(%)
Playing/tricks	35	(18)
Loss of control due to wet surface, loose or broken surface	27	(14)
Travelling too fast downhill or round corners	27	(14)
Fell off—no particular reason	25	(13)
Fell off—bag or clothing caught in wheel	22	(11)
Fell off because of bicycle fault (e.g. brake failure, chain off)	18	(9)
Fell off bumping up or down kerb	12	(6)
Hit debris/obstacle in road	9	(5)
Hit animal	8	(4)
Hit pedestrian	7	(4)
Other	8	(4)
TOTAL	198	

Source: *Hospital Study of Road Accidents* (Transport and Road Research Laboratory, Crowthorne, 1984/5).

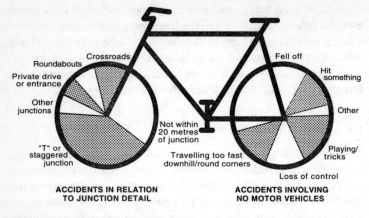

Figure 5.2 Pedal-cyclist casualties
Cycling accidents involving motor vehicles are most commonly associated with road junctions; T-junctions are particularly problematic. When no motor vehicle is involved a wide range of factors have been identified as the primary cause. Most commonly such accidents are caused by cyclists playing or doing tricks on their cycles. *Sources*: Department of Transport, *Road Accidents Great Britain, The Casualty Report* (HMSO, London, 1990), also earlier annual volumes; *Hospital Study of Road Accidents* (Transport and Road Research Laboratory, Crowthorne, 1984/5).

Accidents involving pedestrians

Other than the road-accident statistics recorded on the Stats 19 forms, there is little survey data about accidents between cyclists and pedestrians, and nothing about the precise locations at which these take place. One detailed local study reported little evidence of conflict between pedestrians and cyclists,[21] and the fact that very few pedestrians are killed in collisions with cyclists—only five in 1989—appears to confirm this.[22] Undoubtedly, there are many less-severe collisions between cyclists and pedestrians which are likely to go unreported, and the apprehension pedestrians, particularly the elderly, feel about cyclists on pavements should not be underestimated.

Nature of injuries

The type of injury sustained by cyclists, in particular the body region involved, provides further information towards improving the safety of cyclists. Those regions most frequently reported as being affected are the limbs, with the head being affected in the majority of the remainder.[23] However, when more serious-injury crashes are examined the proportion of head injuries increases. Thompson *et al.* reported that one-third of all bicycle-related injuries treated at an emergency room were head injuries, compared with two-thirds of those requiring admission to hospital.[24] Nixon *et al.* reported that 70 per cent of bicycle-related fatalities were due to head injuries and a further 26 per cent to multiple injuries.[25] However, Mills reported the lower limbs as being the most frequently seriously injured body region, with these injuries often requiring long stays in hospital.[26] Measures to reduce cycle casualties should therefore aim to prevent the most frequent injuries (those of the limbs) as well as those that have the potential to have the most serious outcomes (head injuries).

Cycle paths

In current traffic conditions it is apparent that cycling is a particularly vulnerable form of travel. Somewhat surprisingly, surveys of road accidents in Sweden, West Germany, and the US have shown that the accident-rate per kilometre travelled is approximately three to four times higher on cycle paths compared with motor roads.[27] Conclusions such as these tend to reflect situations where poor crossing arrangements of cycle paths with roads result in the creation of new hazards which tend to cancel out the benefits to cyclists of segregated right-of-way between junctions. It should also be remembered that the figures relate to all severities, that there is a wide variation in levels of accident reporting, and that there are different age-distributions of cyclists in the three countries. There is also some evidence that the dangers of riding on cycle paths can be increased by the greater feeling of safety that cyclists enjoy on exclusive paths, leading some to take less care. Ensuring that cycle paths do in fact make a net positive contribution to cyclists' safety means paying close attention to particular features such as the width of the path, the frequency of junctions with the path and priority arrangements, and inter-visibility of cyclists and drivers. Realization of the potential safety-gains also depends on the adequacy of crossing arrangements, including signing and markings, and the level of maintenance of the path at and near the crossing. Nevertheless, in terms of the more severe types of injury which are the primary concern of bodies promoting cycling for its health and other benefits, it is apparent that the rate is far lower where cyclists can be separated from motor vehicles, as collisions with them are the major source of cyclists' injuries. Reducing motor-vehicle speeds in urban areas and developing integrated cycle networks can also reduce the potential for conflict.

Risk assessment

On the basis of the estimated number of cyclists and the official figures of road deaths, the annual risk of death is about 1 in 14,000 for the 4 million regular cyclists, but the risk of injury is much higher. However, this needs to be seen in perspective. The record of accident statistics in this country shows that, on average, a cyclist can expect to ride over 330,000 kilometres before being seriously injured and 17 million kilometres before being killed. Nevertheless, it is ironic that cyclists, who pose little threat of injury to other road-users, should be so vulnerable to injury from these other users, particularly motorists and lorry-drivers. It is a further irony that the use of cycles is deterred by this threat.

In conclusion, it is salutary to compare the costs of cycle accidents with the costs of their prevention through the provision of safe routes. Table 5.8 has been drawn up on the basis of statistics on road accidents, revised in the light of the under-reporting of injuries cited earlier in this chapter, and 1989 valuations used by the Department of Transport for the costs of these accidents to society. The Table indicates that the cost, if index-linked to 1991, would be over £800 million. Even so, such a calculation on cost-effectiveness takes no account of the indirect benefits such as likely reductions in absenteeism due to improvements in individual health. As these are economic calculations the social benefits of improved public health are also not taken into account. This suggests that the provision of segregated cycle ways, which are very cheap relative to road construction for motor traffic, would be a highly cost-effective form of public investment.

The relative cost of provision for segregated cycle routes as com-

Table 5.8 Costs of accidents among cyclists according to Department of Transport valuations

Injury	No. in 1990 (thousands)	Unit value (£ thousands)	Total (£ millions)
Fatal	0.29	677.7	199.3
Serious	12.40	23.7	293.8
Slight	89.93	2.2	199.7
TOTAL	102.62		692.8

Sources: Department of Transport, *Road Accidents Great Britain: The Casualty Report* (HMSO, London, 1990); P. J. Mills, *Pedal Cycle Accidents—A Hospital Based Study*, TRRL 220 (Transport and Road Research Laboratory, Crowthorne, 1989).

pared to provision for motor traffic can be demonstrated in figures for the cost per mile of such provision. Research has shown provision for motor vehicles ranging from £6.7 million per mile for the M1 widening at Hertfordshire, to £23 million per mile for the Hackney Wick–M11 Link, whilst costs for the Somerstown Cycle Route, London, the Hastingsbury Route, Bedford, and the Stockton Cycle Route were all in the region of £0.1 million per mile.[28]

Air pollution

The effects on fauna and flora of air pollution from industrial sources have attracted considerable attention in the last few decades. Recently, the impacts on human health of air pollution from all sources, including vehicle emissions, have been examined. The subject is relevant to cycling because the physical exertion entailed requires deeper breathing, and its attractions are clearly influenced by people's perception of the quality of the air they breathe; also, and somewhat ironically, cycling has an important contribution to make to a reduction in such air pollution through the transfer from motorized travel to bicycles. Indeed, an objection voiced by many potential cyclists, particularly those who could commute by bicycle, is the extent to which breathing air polluted by chemical components—such as sulphur dioxide, nitrogen oxides, ozone, carbon monoxide, benzene, and airborne particulates—may have adverse effects on their health.

In attempting to determine the effects of air pollution on health a problem arises, as it is not ethical to enter subjects into clinical trials because of the risks to their health. However, there is a growing body of evidence regarding air pollution and standards are now being widely adopted.

Sulphur dioxide

When fossil fuels, especially coal, are burned, the long-stored sulphur is released as sulphur dioxide,[1] and some of this sulphur dioxide is absorbed by plants and animals. In Britain, coal-fired power-stations account for over two-thirds of the non-natural components of these emissions[2]—car exhausts are not a major source. However, because of the increased use of electricity and decline in the use of fossil fuels burned in urban areas, the amount of sulphur dioxide has been falling in European cities. Annual mean levels have decreased generally from within the range of 100–200 $\mu g/m^3$ a decade ago to below 100 $\mu g/m^3$ now, though average levels in some rural areas exceeding 25 $\mu g/m^3$ indicate a spread of such urban pollution,[3] because of the common practice of using high chimneys to disperse emissions. These levels may be contrasted with naturally occurring levels, which are normally below 5 $\mu g/m^3$. The EC guide-line limits on these emissions are 100–150 $\mu g/m^3$ for the 24-hour mean, and 40–60 $\mu g/m^3$ for the annual mean. In London in 1989, the limits were exceeded on nine days at a roadside measuring-station and on seven days at a central London background station.[4] Sulphur-dioxide pollution is measurably highest during periods of stable atmospheric conditions which do not allow for its dispersal at ground level.

Whilst the precise health effects of sulphur dioxide are difficult to measure, high levels can induce breathing problems, such as bronchitis, and asthmatics are particularly badly affected. The most serious health effects occur when it is present in the air at the same time as high levels of particulates, which can adsorb it. In the lungs, the effect of moisture on the inhaled particulates is the formation of sulphuric acid. This lethal combination is thought to be the main cause of death of the 4,000 people who died in the notorious 1952 London smog. Although the World Health Organization (WHO) suggests that the minimum level of sulphur dioxide needed to increase the occurrence of bronchitis is 250 $\mu g/m^3$, short-term reversible changes in the way the lung functions have been observed at much lower levels, particularly in children.[5]

Nitrogen oxides

Nitrogen oxides, by which is generally meant nitric oxide and nitrogen dioxide, result from high-temperature combustion where nitrogen and oxygen in the air combine. It is thought that nitrogen dioxide may trigger biochemical changes at relatively low concentrations, though in animal studies, short-term exposure to low levels have rarely been observed to cause ill effects.[6] On the other hand, long-term exposure at these levels can affect lungs and their functioning. In the case of nitric oxide, one study indicated an increase in airway resistance in healthy persons engaged in light exercise after two hours' exposure to concentrations of about 1,200 µg/m³, which are not uncommon in urban areas.[7]

In Britain, motor-vehicle exhausts are the principal source of nitrogen oxides, being responsible for 45 per cent of emissions. In terms of people in the vicinity of motor vehicles, this is especially important as the gas is expelled close to the ground and thus has a greater local impact. Concentrations fall off quickly away from the curb-side and with height above the pavement,[8] but again adverse effects on health are highest when there is little wind to disperse it at ground level. Levels also vary according to the time of day, the season, and the weather. Highest concentrations are found especially at the roadside during the morning and evening rush-hours in conurbations. In London, annual average concentrations at the top limit of the average urban range around the world of 20–90 µg/m³ have recently been regularly recorded. Occasionally maximum hourly levels exceed 600 µg/m³.[9]

Levels of ozone

Ozone is found naturally in the lower atmosphere, mainly as a result of its diffusion down from the stratosphere. Supplementing this background level, ozone is also produced by a chemical reaction of nitrogen oxides and hydrocarbons combining with sunlight. This leads to the formation of photochemical smog which has adverse effects on health. Motor vehicles provide 45 per cent of nitrogen oxides and 28 per cent of hydrocarbons, and are the major source of the reaction.[10]

No national standards for ambient levels of ozone have been established. Levels of ozone in Britain and on the Continent have been very poorly monitored, but recently its effects have been commonly found in both urban and rural areas, since it is not easily dispersed in air currents. The World Health Organization has set a limit for ozone of the range 0.08–0.10 ppm. However, during the summers of 1976 and 1989 the lower limit for hourly averages was exceeded many times in Britain.[11]

As with the other air pollutants, individuals vary in their reactions to ozone. Goldsmith and Nadel[12] found that broncho-constriction occurs in some people at rest on exposure to an ozone concentration as low as 0.10 ppm. Some changes may occur at even lower concentrations during intense periods of exercise. Exercise performance is impaired after exposure to low levels of ozone in hot weather and it is for this reason that joggers in Los Angeles are advised to stay at home during smog alerts, when maximum hourly ozone concentrations reach 0.30 ppm.

Epidemiological studies have indicated a number of acute effects of ozone and other photochemical oxidants. These include eye, nose, and throat irritation, chest discomfort, coughs, and headaches. Loss of lung efficiency in fit children and young adults has been found with hourly average ozone concentrations in the range of 0.08–0.18 ppm, and in athletic performance in the range of 0.12–0.36 ppm. In addition, an increase in asthmatic attacks and respiratory symptoms has been observed after exposure to similar concentrations.[13] Similar findings were reported in a recent study published in the *Lancet*. The study found that low ozone concentrations, similar to those commonly occurring in urban areas, can increase the bronchial responsiveness to allergen in atopic asthmatic subjects.[14] Somewhat surprisingly, individuals who smoke may be less sensitive to ozone than non-smokers, perhaps because when their lungs come into contact with smoke, the resultant increase in mucous production may have the effect of protecting the lung tissue from irritation by the ozone.[15]

Of all the common air pollutants, except for carbon monoxide, ozone is the one on which there is the most general agreement about ill effects. Studies have been undertaken in the US which attempt to measure the savings in health-costs resulting from reducing various pollutants.[16] The billion dollars which it is estimated could be saved by lowering ozone levels provide a demonstration of the extent to which health is considered to be damaged by this form of pollution. For years this problem was considered to be really serious only in Los Angeles, because of its topography. However, the fact that in 1989 there were fifty-six occasions in central London when average hourly ozone concentrations exceeded 0.08 ppm, the lower limit of the WHO recommended range (0.08–0.10 ppm), and eleven on which the average hourly concentration exceeded the upper limit of 0.10 ppm,[17] suggests that a substantial problem may exist in other locations in the world.

Hydrocarbons and particulates

There are several hundred hydrocarbons and these are formed mainly as a result of the incomplete combustion of organic materials, but are also formed during natural processes. They take many forms and can rearrange to form other hydrocarbons. In an extreme re-arrangement carbon atoms can be released, which combine to form soot particles.

Airborne particulates are made up of a complex mixture of organic and inorganic substances from a variety of sources. Generally they are divided into two groups: coarse particles larger in diameter than 2.5 μm and fine particles smaller than 2.5 μm. The smaller ones include sulphate and nitrate particles, formed in the air from sulphur dioxide and nitrogen oxides combining with combustion particles. The larger particles usually contain materials from natural sources, such as the earth, dust storms, and volcanoes, and non-natural sources such as power-plants, vehicular traffic, and industrial incin-erators. The more important non-natural sources tend to be concen-trated in urban areas with high populations.

Hydrocarbons fall within a broader group called Volatile Organic Compounds (VOCs), including substances such as formaldehyde and benzene. Hydrocarbons can also lodge on particulates which, when inhaled, can cause problems in the lungs. Larger particles are mainly deposited in the nasal passages, while the main proportion of the smaller ones are deposited in the upper airways. During mouth breathing, fine particles less than 2.5 μm in diameter can reach the lungs. The proportion of mouth breathing as opposed to nose breath-ing increases with exercise, such as cycling.

Although about 500 polycyclic aromatic hydrocarbons (PAH) have been found in the air, most measurements have been made on the best known, benzo(a)pyrene (BaP). The natural background level of this is probably nearly zero.[18] However, in major urban areas the levels are now in the range of 1–10 µg/m³. It is thought that there is no safe level for this pollutant.

The inhalation of hydrocarbons, especially benzene, and particulates, is a source of concern because of proven carcinogenicity.[19] Emissions of hydrocarbons from transport sources in Britain, which account for nearly one-third of the total, rose by 60 per cent between 1979 and 1988.[20] Although the catalytic convertors with which new cars purchased from 1993 will have to be fitted will start to reduce these emissions, diesel-powered road-vehicles, whose emissions of particulates are particularly high, will not be subject to this legislative change.

Carbon monoxide

Carbon monoxide is an odourless, colourless gas produced by incomplete combustion of fuel. There are many sources: natural background levels range from between 0.01 and 0.23 µg/m³. However, human activity, such as domestic and industrial fuel use and power-stations are major contributors. In Britain, about 85 per cent of carbon monoxide comes from road transport—the only sector in which it has continued to rise over the last decade—and an even higher proportion in urban areas.[21]

The WHO guideline limit for an 8-hour mean is 10 µg/m³, but in urban areas levels in excess of this have been observed quite frequently in recent years.[22] Most cities have peak-levels coinciding with the morning and evening rush-hours. A safe level is dependent on the carbon-monoxide concentration in inhaled air, the length of exposure, and the ventilation rate.[23]

Excessive intake of carbon monoxide is well known to be injurious to health. Its toxicity results from its affinity for haemoglobin, which carries oxygen round the body. Carbon monoxide binds haemoglobin over 200 times as readily as oxygen, with the result that exposure reduces the amount of oxygen transported around the body. When deprived of oxygen, perception and thinking are impaired and reflexes are slowed down. At very high concentrations death results—witness the number of suicides achieved by extending an exhaust pipe into a sealed car.

Carbon monoxide, once in the body, is not immediately expelled:

Table 6.1 Predicted carboxyhaemoglobin levels for subjects engaged in different types of work

ppm	µg/m³	Exposure time	Predicted % carboxyhaemoglobin level for those engaged in		
			sedentary work	light work	heavy work
100	115.0	15 mins	1.2	2.0	2.8
50	57.0	30 mins	1.1	1.9	2.6
25	29.0	1 hour	1.1	1.7	2.2
10	11.5	8 hours	1.5	1.7	1.7

Source: World Health Organization, *Air Quality Guidelines for Europe*, WHO Regional Publications, European Series 23 (World Health Organization, Copenhagen, 1987).

return to pre-exposure levels takes from two to eight hours. A decreased oxygen-uptake capacity, and the resultant decreased work capacity, has been shown to occur in healthy young adults, starting at a level of 5.0 per cent carboxyhaemoglobin and in some studies, as low as 3.3 to 4.3 per cent (see Table 6.1).[24]

Studies looking at the arrhythmogenic effect of carbon-monoxide exposure in humans have been suggestive in several areas. Nevertheless, a recent study concluded that, although there was a significant increase in amount and severity of ventricular arrhythmia during exercise in response to elevation of carboxyhaemoglobin levels, the clinical importance of this finding in terms of a link between carbon-monoxide exposure and exercise-related arrhythmia possibly leading to sudden death remained to be determined.[25]

However, no major adverse short-term health effects were found in a small sample of cyclists and drivers as a result of the levels of pollution encountered during a test period,[26] though it is worth noting that the carboxyhaemoglobin levels measured in motorists were slightly higher than those in cyclists, a finding reinforced by similar experimental observations.[27] One of the reasons why carbon-monoxide levels are lower on a bicycle than in a car may be because cyclists are generally not sitting stationary behind the exhaust pipes of vehicles in front of them, are breathing in air at least four feet above the roadway surface, and can move ahead of slow or stationary traffic.

Although it is difficult to measure the effects of pollution on health in a precise way, death-rates from asthma have risen by a half in the last ten years, and it is thought that this may be explained by increased levels of pollutants in the air.[28] Clearly the higher the level of pollutants, the greater the likelihood of harmful effects, and cyclists would be well advised to avoid narrow, busy streets where concentrations are highest.

Finally, it may be observed that, while the evidence presented in this chapter suggests, on the whole, that levels of air pollution are not so high as to pose a serious threat to health, there is no doubt that breathing polluted air is unpleasant. Anecdotally, cyclists report feeling more refreshed after a journey on rural rather than urban roads. This is not an inconsequential consideration to take into account in policy formation.

It has been seen that sulphur dioxide is less of a threat than it was, as are some other pollutants, but ozone, volatile organic compounds, and carbon monoxide can have adverse effects. While, as has been noted, new cars purchased after 1993 will have to be fitted with catalytic convertors which will considerably reduce these pollutants, the effect will only be temporary if traffic grows at the rate forecast:[29] air quality in California, where stringent emission-controls have been in force since 1975, has not substantially improved.

Reducing air pollution

It is clear from the research evidence on exercise and health that there are substantial benefits to be gained, both for the individual and for the nation in terms of reduced public health-care costs, if cycling can be restored from its marginal place as a means of transport. Reference has been made earlier to the air-quality guide-lines issued by WHO. A recent United Nations document pointed out that present air-quality values leave little, if any, margin of protection for certain air pollutants.[30] It concluded that millions of Europeans live in areas with air pollution severe enough to cause considerable morbidity and mortality, and recommended that 'immediate abatement and control action should be taken to reduce the severe impact of air pollution in Europe on human health. This action should not be delayed for additional studies'. Transfer from motorized travel to cycles could go some way towards meeting this objective.

Many people commuting into cities travel by car. Many more travel by train or bus which are, in the main, run on diesel fuel which is a major source of pollution. While the transfer of some commuters from private cars on to public transport would lead to a lowering in congestion and air pollution, their transfer to cycling would reduce pollution still further and, as has been seen earlier, is likely to lower health costs. A major reason for this is that air-pollution emissions from cars are much higher on journeys over relatively short distances. For instance, with cold starts, emissions per mile for journeys of two miles or less—easy distances for motorists to transfer to cycling—are 73 per cent, 107 per cent, and 26 per cent higher for hydrocarbons, carbon monoxide, and nitrogen oxide respectively than the average for all car journeys.[31]

No one has yet calculated what reductions in air pollution could be achieved by such a transfer. Some lessons can be learned from a study in the Netherlands town of Gröningen, which has a population of 160,000.[32] Half of its commuters travel by bicycle. Estimates were made of what increases in pollution would occur if most cyclists in that town transferred to car travel at an occupancy of 1.4 per car, leaving 5 per cent still travelling by cycle—a higher percentage than in many parts of Europe. The study also calculated that the annual cost of each transfer, taking account of air-pollution effects, parking, and fuel, was FL519, that is, about £150. It concluded that the amount of carbon monoxide produced would rise from 280 tonnes to 679 tonnes per annum, hydrocarbons from 52 to 126 tonnes per annum, and nitrogen dioxide from 28 to 68 tonnes per annum. Clearly, the transfer of commuters from cars to bicycles would have a considerable influence on lowering air-pollution levels—and by creating this downward spiral might encourage more people to cycle.

A cycle-riding general practitioner some years ago made a calculation about the impact on the environment of his use of the cycle rather than the car:

My car has a standard 2-litre engine and takes in about 1,700 litres of air in covering one mile at a steady 20 mph. (In fact, it is never possible to do a mile like this in London, where a car is for ever braking, accelerating, or idling, so the comparisons which follow are weighted if anything in favour of the car.)

Of the atmosphere's 20.93 per cent oxygen, all but 0.5 per cent is burned in the cylinders, so that in one mile at 30 mph, my car consumes over 340 litres of oxygen while I, seated in it for two minutes, use less than one litre. I ride my bicycle at about 15 mph. To estimate my own oxygen consumption and ventilation when doing this, I enlisted the help of Dr. F. J. Prime at the Brompton Hospital. I rode the bicycle ergometer in his laboratory while he adjusted the load until I felt that I was doing about the same amount of work as I do on the road; this turned out to be approximately 125 watts. My ventilation and metabolic rates measured whilst I was doing this were such that in the four minutes which I would need to cover one mile, I breathe in about 180 litres of air and abstracted from this about seven litres of oxygen. Thus, my car uses almost 50 times the amount of oxygen that I do over the same distance and in addition to this pumps up to 50 litres of carbon monoxide into the air of London, together with hydrocarbons, lead, and some rather unattractive oxides of nitrogen.

To put it another way; at these respective speeds, one litre of oxygen will carry me in my car for five yards, and on my bicycle for 250 yards; and in less than 10 minutes at 30 mph my car will burn up the total daily oxygen output of a fair sized London tree.[33]

There is also the much-overlooked question of pollution by noise, which has many stress- and hearing-related health effects.[34] There is no doubt that this also lowers the quality of the cycle environment. Whilst, surprisingly, there are no surveys of changes in noise-levels over time, the dramatic rise in the volume of traffic on the roads, particularly heavy-goods vehicles, is very likely to have increased this over and above the reductions attributable to improving standards. In this respect, concerns are well founded. In the last ten years alone, the number of registered cars on the roads has risen by 40 per cent and traffic volume has increased by nearly 60 per cent, including a 22 per cent increase in heavy-goods vehicles which are the source of much traffic noise.[35]

The replacement of cars by bicycles would considerably reduce the level of ambient noise. Furthermore, the use of bicycles rather than motor transport could make a substantial contribution to lowering transport-attributable air pollution, in particular greenhouse gases, currently a concern which is rapidly rising to the top of the international political agenda.

From the available evidence, it is clear that effects of air pollution on health depend very much on duration and frequency of exposure.

For the cyclist, the rate and depth of respiration and time of travel must be added as cyclists inhale more air in a given time than the physically inactive car driver. This points to the advantages of cyclists travelling before and after heavy traffic rush-hours, if this is possible, and using less-congested routes on days when pollution levels are high, particularly if they have disorders of the heart or lungs. Moreover, it makes sense for cyclists to try to avoid the direct path of the exhaust fumes from motor vehicles.

The latent demand for cycling

The data on both cycle ownership and use has shown that, because of a highly unsatisfactory environment, cycling plays a small role in the total pattern of personal travel. Indeed, much evidence can be cited to suggest that it has the potential for catering for a much higher proportion of journeys, especially those which are essentially being made on an individual rather than a family basis and, in the case of children, would be made on their own if there was a safe environment for them. Most of these journeys are made on a fairly regular basis— to school, work, shops, and so on.

First, the great majority of the population can cycle: a 1990 survey recorded 99 per cent of men and 87 per cent of women over the age of 15 claiming that they were able to do so.[1] Whilst no national surveys have been carried out on children's ability to cycle, the survey referred to earlier recorded that 90 per cent of both junior-school boys and girls own a bicycle; this would suggest that at least that proportion are able to ride one.[2] However, despite the apparent ability of the vast majority of the population to cycle, there has been a marked decline in cycling.

Table 7.1 shows the very marked increase with age in the proportion of people who have not cycled for many years, and the relatively small difference between men and women in this respect.

Secondly, as noted earlier, bicycle sales have been rising sharply in the last six years and are forecast to rise to 4 million in 1993.[3] With current patterns of growth, it seems likely that ownership will rise to 20 million bicycles in Britain during this decade. Further evidence of prospects in this regard can be drawn from ownership-levels on the Continent: whilst the level in 1985 in Britain was about 24 per 100 per-

Table 7.1 Cycle-riding ability and practice among adults, 1989 (%)

	cannot ride	can ride but have not done so in years	ride sometimes
Gender			
male	1	61	36
female	13	58	29
Age in years			
15–19	7	30	69
20–24	1	47	51
25–44	7	53	37
45–64	10	67	22
65+	9	80	5
All adults	7	59	32

Source: Mintel, *Bicycles* (Mintel International Group, Sept. 1989).

sons, in West Germany it was 74, and in the Netherlands 79.[4] These higher levels on the Continent are not explained by lower levels of car ownership there. Indeed, people in West Germany are about 30 per cent more likely than those in Britain to own a car.[5] Nor is the higher ownership of bicycles there explained by poorer public transport, for the reverse is true—all these Continental countries have a reputation for a high standard of both bus and rail services.

Thirdly, in spite of land use and planning changes in Britain over the years which have led to an extension of the distances that people have to travel to school, shops, recreational facilities, and so on, close examination of the National Travel Survey data reveals that a surprisingly high proportion of journeys are still made over distances which could in theory be conveniently made by cycle.

Table 7.2 shows that half of all journeys are made within a distance-band of about 3 kilometres and three-quarters within an 8-kilometre band. Even if only motorized journeys are considered, it can be seen that a quarter are made within 3 kilometres, and three in five within the 8-kilometre band—a cycling time of less than thirty minutes. Even in today's traffic conditions, where provision for cycling in terms of a dedicated network is extremely rare, a quarter of all cycling journeys are made over distances of 3 to 8 kilometres. In West Germany, two studies have been undertaken to determine the latent demand for cycling. The first estimated that it is possible to transfer 25 to 35 per cent of trips made by car to the bicycle,[6] and the second that, under favourable conditions, up to 50 per cent of school trips, 25 per cent of shopping trips, and 15 per cent of work trips, as well as far more leisure trips, could be made by cycle.[7] More recently a UK study concluded that over 60 per cent of existing trips and over 40 per cent of car journeys were of less than 5 kilometres, and therefore potentially transferable to the cycle.[8]

In the last few decades, land use and location policy has tended to aim to benefit from the internal economies of scale achieved by serving larger population catchments in large but fewer outlets. Advan-

Table 7.2 (a) Proportion of journeys made by cycle, on foot, and by motorized means within different distance-bands as a percentage of the total journeys made by each means of transport

Kilometres	Cycle	Walk	Motorized	All
Less than 1.6	33.4	79.2	7.4	33.5
1.6 to less than 3.2	35.2	16.5	17.2	18.1
3.2 to less than 4.8	14.0	3.0	15.1	10.8
4.8 to less than 8.0	10.6	1.0	20.3	13.3
8.0 to less than 16.0	4.9	0.2	20.2	12.7
16.0 and over	1.1	0.0	18.6	11.6
TOTAL	100.0	100.0	100.0	100.0

Table 7.2 (b) Proportion of journeys made by cycle, on foot, and by motorized means, within different distance-bands as a percentage of the total journeys made within each band

Kilometres	Cycle	Walk	Motorized	All
Less than 1.6	2.4	83.9	3.7	100
1.6 to less than 3.2	4.6	32.2	63.2	100
3.2 to less than 4.8	3.2	10.0	86.8	100
4.8 to less than 8.0	1.9	2.8	95.3	100
8.0 to less than 16.0	0.9	0.6	98.5	100
16.0 and over	0.2	0.1	99.7	100
TOTAL	2.4	35.4	62.2	100

Source: Department of Transport, *National Travel Survey: 1985/86 Report—Part 1: An Analysis of Personal Travel* (HMSO, London, 1988).

tage has been taken of the considerable increase in the availability of cars, allowing those with access to them to travel greater distances to avail themselves of the wider range of choices there. This can be seen, for instance, to be the outcome of policy on school provision which has led to a significant reduction in the number of primary and secondary schools, and therefore the need for the average child to travel further to school.[9] Clearly, if planning and commercial decisions affecting the distances that people have to travel to school, shops, work, leisure facilities, and medical practices took into account their impact on opportunities to travel by cycle, this could lead to a reversal of such policies and a return to a pattern of provision more attuned to local need, enabling more journeys to be made by cycle.

At the same time, people have tended to move to suburbs and rural areas where housing has been built at low densities. This has created life-styles dependent on and encouraging car travel. Again, over time, for the wide variety of social, economic, environmental, and ecological reasons, it may be that this trend will have to be reversed, and this too could lead to wider opportunities for the take-up of cycling as an appropriate means of travel.

Finally, the much higher level of cycle use in countries which make proper provision suggests a further substantial reason for believing that a considerable latent demand for cycling would be released if the deterrents, particularly the fear of a road accident, could be removed. In York and Cambridge in this country, and in many Continental towns, for example in the Netherlands, Denmark, and West Germany, far more journeys are made by cycle: the proportion in Copenhagen is ten times greater than in London, and in small towns, such as Delft and Gröningen, nearly half of all journeys are made in this way.[10]

It is instructive to compare the extent of cycle use in the Netherlands with that in Britain. It is often argued that the Netherlands is a country with few hills, which are clearly a deterrent to cycling. Nevertheless, although there are a great many more settlements in Britain where adverse topography provides a significant deterrent to cycling than there are in the Netherlands, the majority of urban settlements in Britain are in lowland areas with topographical characteristics not so dissimilar to the Netherlands. Although there are differences in terrain, the wide disparity between the figures for the two countries can

Table 7.3 Percentage of all journeys made by cycle in Britain and the Netherlands, according to age-group and gender

	11–15	16–20	21–9	30–59	60–4	65+	All
Male							
Britain	13.4	5.9	2.6	2.1	2.1	2.2	3.2
Netherlands	60.6	47.7	22.2	18.2	21.4	26.4	24.8
Female							
Britain	3.8	1.8	1.3	1.5	1.3	0.5	1.5
Netherlands	60.3	46.9	26.6	30.6	25.1	23.1	31.6

Note: The first two age-groups for the Netherlands cover 12–14 and 15–20 year-olds.
Sources:Department of Transport, *National Travel Survey: 1985/86 Report—Part 1: An Analysis of Personal Travel* (HMSO, London, 1988); *Mobility of the Dutch Population in 1989* (Centraal Bureau voor de Statistiek, Voorburg/Heerlen, 1990).

only be attributed in small measure to this factor. Moreover, the climate in the two countries is not dissimilar.

Table 7.3 compares the proportion of journeys made by cycle by age-group and gender in the two countries. The proportion of journeys made by cycle is greater for all age-groups in the Netherlands, which suggests that if safe provision were made for it the wide-scale benefits identified in the first two sections of this report could be realized in Britain. By looking at the total number of journeys made by cycle in the Netherlands and Britain it can be calculated that twelve times as many journeys are made by bicycle in the Netherlands compared with Britain.

Thus, there are strong grounds for believing that the current patterns of cycling in Britain give a distorted image of the role that cycling could play if the disincentives to its use, particularly the risk of injury, were much reduced, as they could be by adopting the policies and practices on provision for cycling found in the Netherlands.

The role of the individual

The higher volume of traffic has required cyclists to exercise increasing skills in 'reading' the more dangerous environment with its numerous signs and signals, whilst at the same time maintaining balance and keeping a close watch on what is often a poorly maintained road surface. This all demands considerable mental agility. The higher speeds of traffic leave less time for driver and rider to take evasive action in the event of a possible collision. This poses particular problems for children, in view of the fact that their skills are not yet sufficiently developed,[1] and for the elderly cyclists because of their declining skills.[2]

In examining the role of the individual cyclist it should be remembered that few cyclists ride into motor vehicles. Most fatal accidents amongst cyclists occur as a result of being hit by a carelessly driven motor vehicle. Nevertheless, there are several ways by which individuals can counter some of the risk of injury and damage to their health when cycling. These include: improving proficiency and skills in riding; generally taking greater care; maintaining cycles in roadworthy condition; wearing helmets to minimize head injury in the event of accident; improving conspicuity; and wearing face-masks to reduce vehicle-exhaust gases from the air they breathe.

Taking care

Cyclists can take action both with regard to the bicycle that is used and in the skills used when riding it. First, a bicycle needs to be the correct size, as this not only contributes to greater efficiency but also to making steering and general control easier. The top of the handlebars should generally be level with the top of the saddle, which in turn is at the right height when the rider can sit on the saddle with the heel on the pedal at the lowest position and the leg straight, but not stretched. A useful check is whether the toes of both feet can touch the ground when astride the saddle. The bicycle may be fitted with a mirror as an aid to riding but not as a substitute to making a direct visual check, a bell or other audible warning device is also useful. Leather brake blocks are preferable as they perform well in wet and dry conditions and with all types of rim design, although advances in technology have led to the development of synthetic blocks with equally good performance.

Secondly, a bicycle should be kept in roadworthy condition. A survey carried out ten years ago found that one in three of the cycles used by children to go to primary and middle school were in a dangerous condition, and only just over one in three were in good condition.[3] The most common faults were to do with chains, brakes, headsets, tyres, and wheel hubs, most requiring simple adjustment. Clearly, cycles should be checked and maintained on a regular weekly or monthly basis, and an expert service carried out once or twice a year. Figure 8.1 provides a checklist for cyclists to identify potential problems with their cycle.

Thirdly, cyclists should adopt measures which can reduce the risk of their involvement in a road accident. Excellent advice on all aspects of cycling is easily obtained from the Royal Society for the Prevention of Accidents (RoSPA) and from cycling organizations.[4] This obviously includes riding with due care and attention, avoiding main roads where possible; making use of, but not relying on, cycle mirrors; indicating intentions in a decisive way with clear arm-signals when turning, and again where possible, catching the eye of drivers to reinforce that signal; giving a wide berth to parked vehicles; wearing conspicuity aids, such as high-visibility clothes or accessories, and a helmet. Pedestrians should be given priority and cycle bells rung, or a shout given in a considerate way to alert them when necessary. Lights should always be used at night. Furthermore, research has shown that 12 per cent of cyclist fatalities have blood-alcohol levels exceeding 80 mg/100 ml;[5] cyclists should therefore be aware of the particular dangers associated with cycling after drinking.

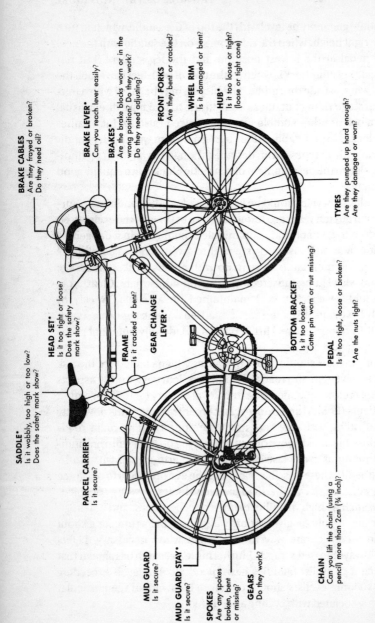

SADDLE*
Is it wobbly, too high or too low?
Does the safety mark show?

HEAD SET*
Is it too tight or loose?
Does the safety
mark show?

BRAKE CABLES
Are they frayed or broken?
Do they need oil?

BRAKE LEVER*
Can you reach lever easily?

BRAKES*
Are the brake blocks worn or in the
wrong position? Do they work?
Do they need adjusting?

FRONT FORKS
Are they bent or cracked?

WHEEL RIM
Is it damaged or bent?

HUB*
Is it too loose or tight?
(loose or tight cone)

FRAME
Is it cracked or bent?

TYRES
Are they pumped up hard enough?
Are they damaged or worn?

**GEAR CHANGE
LEVER***

BOTTOM BRACKET
Is it too loose?
Cotter pin worn or nut missing?

PEDAL
Is it too tight, loose or broken?
*Are the nuts tight?

PARCEL CARRIER*
Is it secure?

MUD GUARD
Is it secure?

MUD GUARD STAY*
Is it secure?

SPOKES
Are any spokes
broken, bent
or missing?

GEARS
Do they work?

CHAIN
Can you lift the chain (using a
pencil) more than 2cm (¾ inch)?

Figure 8.1 Cycle maintenance check points
Ensuring that the bicycle is in a roadworthy condition is one way in which individuals can reduce their risk of accidents. Cycles should be checked and maintained on a regular basis and it is advisable for an expert service to be carried out once or twice a year. Reproduced from the 'Cycleway Tutor's Guide' with the kind permission of RoSPA.

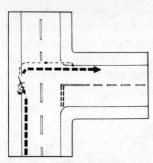

i) Alternative route—major to minor at T-junction or crossroads

- Assess the type of junction ahead. Is the road major or minor? Is it busy? Is there room to stop in the middle of the road?
- Look behind for traffic. How far away is it?
- If you decide it is not safe to move to the centre of the road, continue cycling on the left of the road.
- When you reach the spot where you want to cross, look behind again.
- Give a slowing-down signal.
- Pull into the kerb and dismount. Wheel your bike along the pavement and across the road, using the Green Cross Code.
- Don't forget, always look behind and wait till it is safe before re-starting!
- When turning right from a major to a minor road, it may be possible to stop at the left, then cycle across the road when it is safe. (Diagram i).

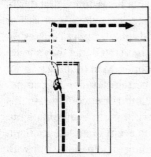

ii) Alternative route—minor to major at T-junction

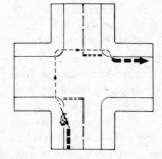

iii) Alternative route—minor to major at crossroads

Walking ---•---   Riding ▬▬▬▬

Figure 8.2 Alternative method of turning right

All cyclists should be aware of defensive cycling techniques that can be adopted where the traffic environment is particularly dangerous. Turning right at a busy junction can pose considerable risks, especially for less confident cyclists; the alternative method of turning right provides a safer option for such cyclists. Reproduced from the 'Cycleway Tutor's Guide' with the kind permission of RoSPA.

Cyclists should be aware of defensive cycling techniques that can be adopted, and motorized traffic should be deferred to when it is clearly appropriate to do so. Cyclists often feel particularly vulnerable when turning right at busy junctions, or when negotiating round-abouts. At these times they can dismount and push their bicycle across the road; full guidance is given in Figure 8.2; this is of particular importance to less-confident cyclists.

Child cyclist training

It needs to be recognized that rules of the road have to be observed and riding skills learned, though it should not be assumed that this in itself will lead to a reduction in the incidence of cycle casualties. For this reason, children in particular should take training courses on basic road-craft. Indeed, the government has stated that they should not cycle in traffic without first having proper cycle training.[6] Given that all other road-users have to attain a certain standard of compe-tence, it does seem sensible that cyclists should be encouraged in this way. Cyclists encounter the same road environment as motorists and are much more vulnerable to injury in the event of a road accident. Children can be taught safe and correct riding to help them cope with the hazards of cycling in traffic.

A training scheme for young cyclists was launched in 1947 by RoSPA, the Cyclists' Touring Club, and the National Cyclists' Union (now the British Cycling Federation). In 1958 the government adopted this as the National Cycling Proficiency Scheme (NCPS) to train children in basic cycle manœuvres, teach them relevant sections of the Highway Code, and to encourage them to maintain their cycles in a roadworthy condition. Since the reorganization of local govern-ment in 1974 the arrangements for training children have been made through the collaboration of local-authority road-safety officers and RoSPA. The scheme is national and voluntary. It involves on average eight to nine hours training for between a quarter and a third of a mil-lion children aged 9 to 12 each year. As a result, well over a half of all cycle-owning children in the country have taken the course. The NCPS has been found to improve basic cycling skills,[7] and to be most effective in the long term when undertaken on minor roads rather than in school playgrounds with roads simulated by plastic cones or painted lines.[8] This form of training has now become the norm.

The NCPS has been criticized for being too much based on instruction and rote learning.[9] Theoretical work in the Netherlands has shown that rules and models are not an appropriate mechanism for teaching certain cycling manœuvres, since children use their own individually determined rules to guide their cycling behaviour for which formal rules cannot be substituted.[10] The implication of this is that a more pro-active form of learning is required.

In the late 1970s a RoSPA working party reviewing all aspects of cyclist training reached similar conclusions and recommended the development of a traffic-education programme for cyclists. The result, *Cycleway*, was published in 1982 as an alternative to the NCPS. It was designed to help children develop a fuller understanding of safer cycling by combining class-room activities involving pupils discussing and solving problems with teaching them to cycle on quiet roads.

Following a government review of road safety in 1987 and changes to the education system, *Cycleway* was revised in conjunction with a 'Cycling Awareness Course', developed by Buckinghamshire County Council. The new course, *Cycleway, the National Course in Cycling Awareness*, was introduced by RoSPA in 1990. It is a practical rider-training course that is intended to actively involve children in the learning process and guide them to work out for themselves the hazards of the road environment and the safe ways to cycle. It is believed that the knowledge, skills, and attitudes acquired this way will be more relevant and long lasting.

Novice cyclists, usually young children, have difficulty in controlling a bicycle and holding its course,[11] and hence are not able to give adequate attention to the secondary processes of perception, speed judgement, and the interpretation of the road environment.[12] In fact, RoSPA does not believe that, as a general rule, children under 9 benefit from a course such as *Cycleway* or the NCPS, but that basic training in cycle-handling and road-sense can play a useful supporting role to later, more-comprehensive programmes. Therefore the minimum age for children to take a training course is normally 9 or 10 years.

Some local authorities do conduct basic training for 7 and 8 year-olds, concentrating on informing parents of potential dangers on the road and their responsibilities as parents and motorists, competent bicycle handling, and basic bicycle safety checks. Such schemes do play a valuable role provided that they do not encourage under-nines to use the road unsupervised, do not give a false sense of security to children and their parents, and do not diminish efforts to train older and more receptive children.

A system of grades for cyclist training to enable young cyclists to increase their skill by progressing from one grade to the next has been proposed,[13] and there has, in fact, been a Silver and Advanced level of the NCPS since the 1970s. They have been rarely used, however, largely due to a lack of school and local-authority resources, school time, and interest from older children. To be effective such a system would need to reflect the reasons for, and type of, cycling by older children, and would require an increase in the resources available for training.

RoSPA has proposed to the National Curriculum PE Working Group that basic cycling and road-craft be included in the Physical Education Curriculum. This would convey considerable educational, health, and accident-prevention advantages. Given the existence of well-developed training schemes it would be relatively easy and inexpensive to implement, and would offer numerous opportunities for establishing clear and strong cross-curricular links between Physical Education and the core subjects (English, Mathematics, and Science) and Technology at the very least.

As local authorities have the statutory responsibility for road safety for all road-users, and as there has been a considerable growth in sales of cycles among adults, there seems to be a strong case for introducing cycle training for them as well. Children can also learn road skills by cycling with their parents, as they do by walking with their parents. Indeed, it has been suggested that there may be some link between the low use of cycles by adults and the relatively high cycle-accident rate among children.[14]

Training for children in cycling safety is clearly a priority area. However, two cautionary notes need to be sounded about improving cycling skills, particularly among children. First, participation in training schemes tends to encourage more frequent cycle use,[15] and therefore exposure to the relatively high risk of injury among cyclists in road accidents. Secondly, the fact that children have passed the cycle test may give them and their parents a false sense of security, in that the impression may be gained that, having passed the test, the children will be safe to cycle on main roads. Passing a training course is a first step, not an end-result, and it is essential for parents to provide continuous help and guidance to their children.

These two factors, in combination, may indeed account for the fact that improvement of cycling skills through the medium of the NCPS has not been shown to have had a demonstrable effect on reducing casualties.[16]

Cycle helmets

People who lose control of their bicycle when travelling at speeds in excess of 20 kph, and who then hit their head on something solid, are almost certain to die.[17] Indeed, head injury has been found to be the primary or contributory cause of death in about two-thirds of fatalities among cyclists.[18] Although head injuries account for a much higher proportion of cyclists' deaths than that of other road-user groups,[19] this type of injury is also common among motorists and pedestrians, who do not normally wear any form of head protection, and even among motor-cyclists for whom the wearing of crash-helmets is compulsory. The higher proportion of head injuries in the fatal and serious accidents involving cyclists is the primary justification for the claims that their fatality-rate could be sharply reduced by the wearing of safety helmets.[20]

In order to assess the degree of protection afforded by cycle helmets the nature of head injury needs to be understood. The human brain has the consistency of a jelly and is surrounded by fluid within the skull. Head injuries occur when the head hits an object or a blow hits the head, causing the brain to move within its surrounding fluid and hit the inside of the skull. Functional or structural damage can occur to nerve fibres that link different parts of the brain, to brain cells which can be killed, and to the supporting tissue of the brain. The degree of damage suffered relates to the force of the deceleration or acceleration caused by the accident. With high-speed impacts the brain can be so badly damaged that death occurs. With lower decelerations the damage is less, so that subjects may live but remain in a coma, or with lesser forces awaken with serious defects in brain function. With smaller forces a period of unconsciousness will be followed by apparently complete recovery. However, the Board of Science and Education Working Party on Boxing found that blows to the head which caused as little as five minutes unconsciousness caused permanent damage to the brain which could subsequently be detected by special test methods.[21] In addition, some authorities believe that certain cases of senile dementia may be related to previous minor head injuries, and around 5 per cent of those suffering head injuries subsequently develop epilepsy.[22]

Head injuries may involve damage to blood vessels that pass to and from the brain within the skull. Bleeding inside the skull can cause compression of the brain, which may be fatal or result in permanent brain damage even though the force causing the head injury is apparently trivial. With more severe injuries, the skull itself may be fractured; whilst this does not affect the immediate management of the patient, displaced parts of the skull and/or fractures of the base of the skull are usually associated with more severe brain damage.

In the most severe accidents, death will frequently result from other bodily injuries which helmets clearly do not prevent, although it has been suggested that helmet wearing might prevent death for a third of accidents which are presently fatal.[23] Though death by accident is tragic, it is important to concentrate on non-lethal head injuries with serious consequences, since crash-helmets could have the greatest potential benefit with this type of injury.

Protection from wearing cycle helmets

Bicycle helmets are designed to protect cyclists by cushioning their heads from the impact of a fall. The shock is absorbed by a thick, crushable layer of expanded polystyrene. This reduces the force of the impact before it reaches the head. Many helmets have a hard outer shell which spreads the energy from a blow and protects the inner liner. Other, lighter helmets, just have the protective liner of expanded polystyrene and a mesh cover to stop it being damaged. It is therefore unlikely that this type of helmet would provide protection from sharp objects. In marked contrast to motor-cycle helmets, any impact, including simply dropping the helmet on the pavement, causes the polystyrene liner to lose its effectiveness. Thus, the helmet must be replaced even if there is no visible damage.

Specifications for cycle helmets are laid down in the British Standard (BS6863). The Standard ensures that the helmet absorbs sufficient impact to be useful and does not impair any of the senses of the wearer. A European standard is currently being developed, which would apply throughout the EC.

Arguments for the generalized use of cycle helmets

The Royal Society for the Prevention of Accidents recommends that cyclists wear a helmet as one way of protecting themselves. The medical community too is generally in favour, as it has been with other road-safety measures. For example, its support was influential in the decision to make seat-belt wearing mandatory in Britain.

Advocates of cycle helmets argue that the majority of serious cycle accidents do not involve collisions with motor vehicles but are caused by cyclists falling off after losing control or encountering a road hazard. One study of bicycle accidents among children under 12 years old showed that most occurred as a result of playing or doing tricks, and secondly as a result of travelling too fast and subsequently losing control.[24] It is for this reason that children are particularly advised to wear helmets.

The relatively low level of cycle-helmet usage has precluded a mass data-based scientific evaluation of the effectiveness of helmet-wearing in reducing injury and death. As a result, proponents of helmet wearing have only been able to substantiate their claims by localized studies from which only limited conclusions can be drawn.[25]

The most widely quoted study was conducted at five major hospitals in the Seattle area of the US. It found that cyclists with helmets had an 85 per cent reduction in their risk of head injury and an 88 per cent reduction in their risk of brain injury.[26] It was concluded that 'bicycle safety helmets are highly effective in preventing head injury'. In Australia, an association between the use of cycle helmets and the reduction in the severity of injury was also found in a postal survey of cyclists.[27] The authors claimed that the study was the first to make a direct comparison of cyclists wearing helmets and those not wearing them, and that their results actually underestimated the association due to their inability to include the most severe accidents in the survey. It was estimated that 90 per cent of deaths by head injury would be prevented by hard-shelled helmets with a complete inner liner. In the UK, Mills conducted a hospital-based study of 776 cyclist casualties, concluding that the use of protective headgear would reduce the number and severity of injuries to cyclists.[28]

While these research findings appear to demonstrate clear advantages in the use of cycle helmets, it should be noted that the sample size of the studies was small. The Seattle study was restricted to 235 incidents of head injury and the Australian study to 197 injuries. It should also be noted that as a case-controlled study, the Seattle research did not distinguish the cycling behaviour of people wearing helmets from those who don't. It is not unreasonable to hypothesize that people wearing helmets, having a greater regard for safety, cycle more safely than those who do not. Although these studies provide useful preliminary data, further research is required in order that more authoritative recommendations can be made.

Deterrents to wearing cycle helmets

There are a number of reasons why most cyclists do not wear helmets. Many cyclists cite discomfort as a reason, although helmets that weigh around a quarter of a pound cannot be said to be a hindrance. On the whole, discomfort stems from unfamiliarity and hence is likely to be short-term. However, the tests referred to above showed that, in general, the lighter the helmet the less shielding it gave. The reason for this is that the denser and thicker the expanded polystyrene liner, the more chance there is of the helmet providing protection. The better helmets tend to weigh around half a pound, and are thus more uncomfortable. Another cause of discomfort is the chin-strap for, to be effective, this must be under tension. Hard-shell helmets also diminish head ventilation and increase head surface-temperature, thus preventing surplus-heat removal, particularly from the crown of the head. It has been estimated that in low temperatures up to one-third of the total heat production may be lost through the head.[29] Much anecdotal evidence suggests that excessive heat is a particular problem with hard helmets, especially in warm weather, and this could be even more uncomfortable for cyclists wearing masks. Nevertheless, one study has found that wearing a helmet does not alter thermal balance.[30]

A further drawback is the inconvenience for cyclists of having to carry around a helmet. A cyclist already has to carry such accessories as lights, a pump, and a reflective sash and trouser-clips. A helmet is heavier and more bulky than all of these put together, and cannot easily be put away in an office drawer or case as can these other items. Because of its value, in the range £20 to £50, it is a great attraction to a thief. Indeed, the high cost of an effective cycle helmet is in itself a deterrent to its purchase and use. At a cost of up to £50, a significant proportion of the price of an average bicycle, they can hardly be said to be within every cyclist's reach.

Children: a separate issue?

There has been more pressure for children to wear helmets than there has been for adults. Children are considered to be too young to take responsibility for accident prevention, and indeed, it has been argued that 'encouraging children to wear helmets is probably the single most important intervention that could be made to reduce the likelihood of serious injury to child bicyclists'.[31] Since injuries of child cyclists are more likely than those of adult cyclists to occur without collision with a motor vehicle, and smaller children have softer bones, it is argued that cycle helmets would contribute more to reducing head injuries in the young.

In recent years BMX bicycles have been widely used by children. They are intended for off-the-road use, and can encourage dangerous behaviour as they are specifically designed to enable them to be used for stunts.[32] Clearly, helmets could prevent head injuries among this type of cycle user as well as those who use the currently more fashionable mountain bikes off the road, since falls from these bikes are more common than when using cycles on the roads.[33] As noted earlier, the cycle helmet provides greater protection for those accidents which do not involve collisions with motor vehicles.

The problem of the high cost of cycle helmets could be a deterrent during childhood, as a change of helmet is likely to be needed as the head increases in size: there are a variety of sizes, and an appropriate one is required to fit very snugly in order to be effective.[34] It is for this reason that the Road Safety Unit of one local authority enlisted the support of schools and youth organizations to lower the cost of safety helmets for children through bulk-purchase agreements, and has been successful in encouraging other local authorities to act in the same way.[35] In addition, children are more likely to be concerned about the image portrayed by wearing a helmet rather than its function:[36] substantial negative peer-group pressure has been found to militate against children wearing them.[37] The wearing of cycle helmets could be encouraged in school-safety classes and community traffic-safety programmes, but the presentation has to be sensitive to current perceptions of the helmet. It would be easier if cycle helmets were not perceived by children to be an item with a negative or 'sissy' image. Indeed, helmets could be more attractively designed, in particular with the teenage market in mind. In this connection, the media have a role to play in showing children wearing helmets. A recent initiative from the government to encourage children to wear cycle helmets has adopted the slogan *Tough Nuts are Hard To Crack*, although it is not possible to make an immediate judgement about the effectiveness of this campaign.

The issue of cycle helmets for children includes the use of headgear for very young children on the back of adult bicycles. One study of cycle injuries to under-5 year-olds in California found that 28 per cent of injuries occurred where bicycle-mounted child-seats were used, 65 per cent of injuries involved the head, and 29 per cent of these injuries were serious. The authors recommend helmets for children carried on adult bikes.[38]

There is a danger of parents viewing the purchase of helmets for their children as a panacea, feeling that they have fulfilled their responsibility for the child's safety; this may also be apparent in encouraging their children to take the NCPS. Such an attitude, without more sustained commitment by parents, might encourage a feeling of false complacency and therefore greater risk of accidents. Parents should pay continuing attention to their child's safety to ensure that safe bicycle-riding is maintained.

Mandatory wearing of helmets

The wearing of cycle helmets has recently become mandatory in two states in Australia and in a district of one state in the US. In New South Wales, both child and adult cyclists not wearing safety helmets face a $32 on-the-spot fine. It has been argued that legislation should be introduced to make helmet-wearing mandatory in the UK. However, the wearing of cycle helmets is only one element of the available measures to enhance cyclists' safety. Department of Transport figures show that 95 per cent of cycle fatalities and 90 per cent of serious injuries occur as a result of motor vehicles; it is therefore vital that the debate on the use of cycle helmets should not obscure more important areas of road safety, which involve action on behalf of motorists, road planners, and policy-makers.

It may be many years before all towns and cities have safe, adequately designed cycle networks. Until then, government could play an important role in carrying out research to establish the effectiveness of helmets in general. Provisional data suggests that good-quality helmets may be a useful short-term measure to reduce the severity of some types of cycle injury, but this needs to be confirmed by further research.

Legislation may distract attention from more effective means of reducing the number and severity of cycle accidents, such as lowering the speed of motor vehicles by traffic-calming, improving the conduct of drivers, especially by more effective enforcement of drink-driving legislation, the separation of bicycles and motor vehicles, and better visibility. The proportion of cyclists wearing a helmet at present is so low that a major and expensive enforcement programme would be needed if there were to be legislation making the wearing of helmets mandatory. Public funding of a campaign for the use of cycle helmets is also likely to draw funding away from these other measures which have greater scope for reducing cycle accidents. It is towards these more efficient ways of preventing accidents that resources should be concentrated.

A central argument for legislation enforcing the use of cycle helmets is that society usually has to pay the medical costs of head injuries suffered by cyclists. The cost of health-care, the loss of working time, and the demands on friends and relatives can have a substantial economic and social impact. However, head injuries are a common cause of death and morbidity, occurring frequently in car drivers and pedestrians. It is therefore questionable why cyclists are being singled out to wear helmets rather than other non-helmeted road-users who have higher risks that also result in a high cost to society.[39] Whilst the universal wearing of cycle helmets may lead to a reduction in injuries needing hospital care, a more dramatic reduction could be achieved by forms of intervention that require action by motorists.

As discussed earlier, a cycle helmet is expensive and many cyclists could find it difficult to afford one. Were cycle helmets to become compulsory this could act as a financial deterrent to cycling. It would be ironic if a measure designed to protect cyclists in fact resulted in fewer cyclists taking to the road.

It has been seen that resources are almost certainly better directed towards the prevention of accidents rather than the limitation of the damage caused by them. The introduction of mandatory wearing of cycle helmets shifts responsibility for the safety of cyclists to the cyclists themselves, despite the fact that they are far more vulnerable and unable to control potentially dangerous situations. It seems more appropriate that responsibility should be borne by those causing the injuries, namely drivers of motor vehicles. Few cyclists ride into motor vehicles. Most fatal accidents among cyclists occur as a result of being hit by a carelessly driven motor vehicle. Nevertheless, a certain number of accidents will be caused by carelessly ridden bicycles, or indeed motorists may have no time to take avoiding action due to poor visibility. One study which sought to identify the 'responsibility' for cycle–motor-vehicle collisions found that almost all children under 15 had cyclist-'responsible' accidents. Nevertheless, almost two-thirds of adult cyclists (age 20 and over) were in accidents where the motorist was 'responsible'.[40]

The question of cycle helmets goes to the heart of policy-making for cyclists. Sooner rather than later it should be realized that the route to encouraging cycling and making it safer lies in the provision of safe cycling networks, enforced lower speed-limits, and in changing the attitudes and behaviour of drivers rather than cyclists.

Conspicuity aids

Speed affects visual perception, especially at night, and faster travel requires more light for safety. Indeed, light from the moon may be sufficient for walking, but is insufficient for motorway driving. Poor visibility of cyclists is a major causal factor of bicycle accidents on public roads. This is not just during twilight and night-time riding, but also during the daytime when 78 per cent of injuries involving adult cyclists occur, and over 90 per cent of those involving child cyclists.[41] The relatively small image of a bicycle compared to other vehicles on the road, and the fact that cyclists are usually on the near-side of the road mean that they are often on the periphery of a driver's vision or obscured by roadside objects or other vehicles. For these reasons, an important way of reducing accidents involving cyclists is to improve their conspicuity, which can be achieved through two main methods.

First, there are lighting systems and reflectors which are attached to the bicycle itself. Such lights are not primarily designed to help a cyclist see his or her way in the dark, nor even to reveal obstructions or pot-holes on unlit roads; rather they are an aid to other road-users, making cyclists more conspicuous. However, these are not necessarily effective, as cyclists often use them when batteries need replacing or the lights are obscured, for instance by a basket or by clothing,[42] and indeed, the rear red lens cuts 75 per cent of the light output.[43] Unlike cycle helmets, the use of lights is mandatory. The legislation requires that between sunset and sunrise, and when visibility is seriously reduced, all cyclists must have a white front light, a red rear light, and a red rear reflector. This law has not been well enforced: in 1984, a survey in four towns in Britain showed that only three-quarters of cyclists had both lights and that 9 per cent had neither.[44]

The large majority of cyclists use battery lights, despite their proneness to theft and the fact that batteries are relatively expensive. The alternative is dynamo lighting which is usually driven by friction of the dynamo on the tyre, causing a slight drag. Although dynamos are now being developed with some storage capacity, the output of the lamp on most of them is dependent on the speed of the bicycle, so that when the bicycle is at a standstill there is no light, and this can be a serious drawback. The absence of a light for right-hand turns, involving a cyclist waiting in the centre of the road until there is a break in the oncoming traffic, poses a risk for cyclists who are then less likely to be seen by following or oncoming traffic. In fact, such a manœuvre without lights at night-time is illegal under the Road Vehicle Lighting Regulations 1989. A proportion of the 11 per cent of accidents involving cyclists which occur when they are turning or waiting to turn[45] may be accounted for by this particular problem. A further problem with dynamo lights is that they may be slightly affected by rain or snow. Nevertheless, tests have shown that cycle lights are detectable at large distances, even against high levels of glare, as long as batteries are not low.[46]

The second aid to conspicuity is high-visibility clothing. A large variety of reflective or fluorescent items is available on the market, ranging from cycling shoes with fluorescent stripes and reflective trouser-clips to reflective head-bands and hats. However, the survey referred to earlier recorded that only 8 per cent of cyclists wore high-visibility clothing in the daytime, and only 10 per cent at night-time,[47] though the impact of recent publicity on this subject is likely to have led to an increase in this proportion.[48]

The most comprehensive study of the effectiveness of reflective clothing evaluated the visibility of a range of conspicuity aids.[49] The distance from which a cyclist is visible and the berth given by overtaking motorists was tested for each type of aid. It was found that cyclists wearing clothing covering a larger body-area and made of material with a higher luminance factor were detected from a greater distance and given a larger berth. Although a reflective hat does not cover a large body-area it performed very well, since it receives direct overhead light during daytime. Although less effective at this time, arm-bands and sashes (Sam Browne belts), because of their diagonal position, stand out from the rest of the road environment and hence catch the eye.

All new bicycles (except certain specialized types) supplied in the UK must comply with the British Standard BS6102, part 1. Amongst other things, this standard requires that bicycles are fitted with front, rear, pedal, and spoke reflectors (or reflective tyres) at the point of sale. Reflectors are also frequently added to carriers and panniers. These may be of marginal use, as the area they cover is so small that the benefit has been found to represent only a fraction of that of reflective clothing.[50] The most effective items in terms of attracting attention are reflectors attached to spokes and white-wall tyres, since they revolve when cycling and therefore catch the eye. They are visible when the bicycle is seen in profile, which is when many accidents occur, for example, when a cyclist is coming out of a side road. Thus, they can contribute to reducing accidents. Pedal reflectors are also particularly effective as they move up and down as the cyclist pedals. Spacers or flags—plastic bars with reflective discs at their end—can be fitted to the frame or rear carrying-rack of bicycles, as they encourage drivers to give cyclists a wider berth.[51]

As ways of improving road safety, conspicuity aids, both lights and reflective material, serve different purposes to cycle helmets. Whereas cycle helmets are intended to reduce the severity of injuries caused by accidents, conspicuity aids are intended to give earlier warning of the presence of a cyclist and thereby reduce the chances of, or prevent, collisions with other vehicles in the first place. In this sense, they represent a more preventative approach to road safety than helmets. However, the arguments rehearsed in the section on helmets about who is responsible for cyclists' safety still apply.

Whilst there is no direct evidence that conspicuity aids reduce the incidence of accidents involving cyclists, there is a prima facie case for believing that they do improve road safety, since lights and reflective clothing clearly help motorists to see cyclists from a greater distance and hence react sooner. Obviously, the more powerful the lamp, the more fluorescent the clothing, and the larger the area it covers, the more effective the conspicuity aid will be. It is a matter of personal choice for individual cyclists as to the extent to which they attempt to make themselves visible.

Once again, the implication of the widespread use of conspicuity aids is that it is the responsibility of cyclists to make sure that they are seen by drivers. If drivers come to believe that it is the responsibility of cyclists to attract their attention, they may become even less vigilant on the roads. Moreover, the theory of risk compensation suggests that motorists will adjust to the reduction in the risk of accidents caused by an increase in the use of conspicuity aids by driving marginally faster, thereby maintaining their risk threshold.[52]

The obvious extension of the argument for more widespread use of conspicuity aids by cyclists is that if they substantially reduce the chances of accidents then all pedestrians would also benefit from their use. If all pedestrians walking after dusk were to wear high-visibility jackets and hats and to have front and rear lights strapped round their waists the chances of pedestrians or cyclists suddenly coming into vision would be minimized, and this would therefore contribute to accident prevention. It must be asked whether this is a reasonable approach to road safety and whether it would be more appropriate if responsibility for accident-prevention was taken by those who are the primary cause of the danger, namely those driving motorized vehicles.

Face-masks

An earlier chapter has reviewed the evidence on the impact of polluted air on the health of cyclists. Certain levels of air pollutants are known to narrow and damage the linings of the air-passages such as the nose, throat, and lungs, and those exposed to pollution are more likely to get respiratory infections and have other medical conditions exacerbated. Clearly the damage caused depends on the levels of pollution, the amount of time spent breathing the air, and on the proximity to the primary sources of the pollution. In both these respects cyclists could be considered to be more at risk than the general population.

Protection against certain air pollutants can be gained if cyclists wear a mask. There are two varieties. The cheapest consists of a simple dust filter that traps particulates, the major source of which, as has been noted, is from diesel exhausts. The other is designed to prevent particulates, hydrocarbons, nitrogen dioxide, nitrogen oxide, sulphur dioxide, and ozone from reaching the lungs. Their efficiency is dependent on how well the mask fits over the face. However, it should be noted that all road-users breathe the same air. Indeed, motorists are to some extent more at risk, as in stationary traffic or in queues polluted air is drawn through the car's ventilation system, whereas cyclists can more easily avoid stopping behind exhaust pipes.

Some masks are designed to be worn for a limited time and then thrown away. Others have washable bodies and replaceable filters. If the activated charcoal filter does not fit perfectly, inhaled air takes the easiest possible route and gets into the lungs round the side of the filter. One type of mask has a one-way valve to help remove exhaled air more quickly, but it has not yet been officially approved.

There are various problems with the use of masks. First, none of the masks available filter out carbon monoxide, which, as has been seen, is one of the most common and harmful pollutants. Secondly, they are uncomfortable and really not very pleasant to wear, and become less comfortable at faster cycling speeds—which is when they are potentially more effective since inhalation is deeper at these times. Thirdly, if they are worn for too long wearers may actually be doing themselves more harm than good, as masks can desorb pollutants if filters are not changed regularly. A wearer could then breathe in chemicals previously absorbed by the filter, causing a greater inhalation of pollutants than without a mask.[53] Fourthly, people have different-shaped faces but the mask is designed for the 'average, normal face'.[54] Finally, a mask and a helmet, which it has been noted can lead to overheating of the head, may cause cumulative discomfort.

Some cyclists wear masks and some do not. It is clear that those who have problems with their breathing and wish to cycle in polluted urban areas should wear masks and should avoid exercise at times of the day when the air is highly polluted and there is little wind-movement to dispel the pollutants. Cycle couriers who are exposed for substantial lengths of time, and anybody cycling on a route heavily used by lorries and thus exposed to high concentrations of particulates, should wear a mask.[55] From the evidence on air pollution there would seem to be little need to wear them on lightly trafficked suburban streets, particularly if route and time of day can be chosen to avoid streets when they are likely to be polluted. On the other hand, as a gesture towards altering public attitudes cyclists wearing masks draw attention to the problem of air pollution. Although masks are recommended as a means of protection against heavily polluted areas, it is obvious that reducing air pollution is the most appropriate and effective solution to this problem.

It could perhaps be suggested that better methods can be used by individuals to reduce the health-and-safety risks of cycling than by taking the precautions described in this chapter. Campaigning for local authorities to adopt lower speed-limits and traffic-calming, to undertake better road maintenance and provide cycle networks, and for central government to alert motorists to the effects of their behaviour on cyclists and in particular in discouraging cyclists, and on the setting of stricter standards on vehicle-exhaust emissions, could be more effective in promoting the health-and-safety interests and rights of cyclists.

In turn, this points to two conclusions: first, that it is dangerous to pass all responsibility for road safety on to those who are most vulnerable. Rather, it is those who are the source of most of the danger, the motor-vehicle drivers, and those in a position to alter the traffic environment, for instance through the medium of 'traffic-calming', who should have the primary responsibility for ensuring cyclists' safety. Secondly, it could be argued that it is immoral to allow people, especially children, to have bicycles and to encourage them to acquire skills to use them, but then to leave them to exercise these skills in environments that can be highly dangerous.

Public policy and practice

Anyone given the task of devising a strategy aimed at ordering the various mechanized methods of transport according to the social and environmental impacts they impose in use, and at promoting patterns of travel conducive to public health, would have to conclude that cycling is the method deserving the highest priority. Yet the relatively low use of cycles on the roads of Britain, despite annual sales reaching levels similar to those of cars, seems to have led transport policy-makers to overlook to a great extent the benefits that could be derived from encouraging more cycling. Ironically, people who cycle—and therefore whose actions are beneficial both to their own health and to the wider public health—do so in an environment which has been rendered less and less pleasant by traffic.

Current policy on cycling

Current transport policy is focused on accommodating life-styles dependent on increased ownership and use of cars. It has been formulated in the belief that growth in car use and expansion of the road network are indicators of progress and of higher standards of living. In many respects, the outcome has been prejudicial to public health, not least in terms of road accidents and the fear and anxiety associated with the risk of them occurring.

Nevertheless, government has taken a growing interest in cycling, particularly in its safety aspects. Many local-transport notes and traffic-advisory leaflets with guidance and technical advice on cycling have been produced in the last few years. Regional Cycling Officers have been appointed to ensure that the needs of cyclists are fully considered when trunk roads are designed or improved, and several local authorities now have cycling officers. In inviting submissions for grants from central government, local authorities have been informed that expenditure on provision for the needs of cyclists will be eligible, but the proposals must be aimed at reducing accidents and are for roads of more than local importance.[1] The Department of Transport have also committed themselves to institute safety audits for new roads, which will set out procedures for checking new road schemes and 'engineering-out' potential accident problems before the scheme is opened.[2]

Since the 1977 Transport White Paper which proposed funding for local cycling schemes, an increasing number of authorities have sought to cater for cycling. Half of the local-authority submissions for central-government funding for 1989 made specific reference to plans for improving facilities for cycling. In all, since 1978 about thirty 'innovative' projects have been promoted jointly by the Department of Transport and certain local authorities. Most of these have been isolated facilities such as new types of signalled cycle crossings or special arrangements at roundabouts. However, five of these, first announced in 1984, have been larger in scale, with some attempt to form a network. This was most extensive in the case of the Greater Nottingham Cycle Route Network, officially completed in the autumn of 1990. Despite various problems, and being much more limited in scope than some comparable Continental special cycling projects, such as the Delft network in the Netherlands, they have proven a most important commitment. Close monitoring of such projects has helped to provide many useful lessons for future efforts.

Most recently the Department of Transport has backed the 'Feet First / A Step Ahead' campaign promoted by the lobby group Transport 2000. Fifteen schemes, that may be adopted nation-wide, have been launched to give pedestrians, cyclists, and buses priority over cars and lorries. In addition, many local authorities have made very significant progress on cycle schemes without Department of Transport assistance. These include the extensive development of off-highway cycle-ways, mostly on disused railways in areas like Lothian Region in Scotland. The most important of these local authority initiatives was the work of the Greater London Cycling Project Team from 1981 until the abolition of the Greater London Council in 1986. In subsequent years it became much harder to sustain this momentum in more than a handful of London boroughs. However, in 1990, the minister with responsibility for this policy issue at the time welcomed 'in principle' a proposal by the cycling lobby for a thousand miles of strategic cycle network for London.[3]

Recent legislation allows local authorities to introduce a wide range of traffic-calming techniques and will soon permit them to create '20 mph zones' in residential areas. Furthermore, recent reviews of speed-limits that resisted calls for an increase in the motorway speed-limit have identified two detailed areas where further work is needed. The Secretary of State for Transport has asked officials to review the criteria which local authorities are required to apply when setting a local speed-limit, and the County Surveyors' Society and the Department of Transport will be identifying measures which can constrain vehicle speeds through villages and moderate driver behaviour. However, it can be argued that traffic-calming measures are of more limited value for cyclists without wider changes in town-planning and traffic-management policies and, at the more detailed level, if designed without careful regard for cyclists' safety and convenience.[4] Detailed guidance on different methods of traffic-calming is available;[5] in particular, such guidance outlines the design considerations necessary for the different measures to be of benefit to cyclists. Overall, for such schemes to be of advantage to cyclists, a reordering of priorities in favour of pedestrians and cyclists should be the common aim as has been the case on the European mainland.

Cyclists and pedestrians will benefit too from the reduction in air pollution resulting from the inclusion of the additional check on exhaust emissions under the annual MoT test, and the requirement that all new cars be fitted with catalytic converters from 1993. As part of a reform of the Public Utilities Street Works Act 1950 (PUSWA), changes in the law requiring utilities to have sole responsibility for making good road surfaces which they have dug up is likely to improve road surfaces that cyclists have to traverse.

However, a compilation of evidence on factors affecting cycle provision, its attractions, and therefore its use as a highly appropriate mode for a much higher proportion of the journeys that people now make, could lead to a view that the need to cater for cycling is, to say the least, not taken very seriously. Nor would this be surprising. Changes in the extent of use of cycles poses a dilemma for government. Whilst it acknowledges that 'cycling is a healthy and environmentally-friendly method of travel and that cyclists have as much right to use the roads as anyone else',[6] cycling remains one of the least safe modes of transport and 'it cannot be the Department's role simply to encourage people to cycle'.[7] The evidence suggests an unintentional outcome of policy, namely that it is preferable for cycling to be discouraged.

Only 1 to 2 per cent of civil servants in the Department of Transport deal with cycling, even on a part-time basis.[8] Moreover, their effectiveness in promoting cycling is questionable, as cycling represents only a small part of their total work-load and as their sole focus of interest is in its safety aspects. Since the reorganization of the Transport and Road Research Laboratory—the research wing of the Department of Transport—research on cycling has been much reduced and is exclusively focused on safety aspects.

The recently published guide to the Department's activity, though referring to its role as 'facilitating movement', does not allude to cycling in the section on transport and the economy,[9] perhaps because the sums involved are so small that they are not seen to be worth recording. The only time that cycling is referred to is under the heading of 'traffic management' where it is simply included in the list of ways of travelling to work or school. By contrast, in the US the promotion of cycling is part of Federal transportation policy: planners and engineers are encouraged to accommodate the bicycle in designing transport facilities in urban and suburban areas.[10]

Symptomatic too of the Department of Transport's attitudes is the oversight of cycling in such statements as 'the environmental effects of road transport—noise, community severance, vibration, visual intrusion and fumes—are common to all [sic] modes'.[11] A recent departmental Library Bulletin listed an important report on the bicycle[12] under the section on 'recreation/tourism/sport' rather than more obviously under a transport heading.

The preface to the most-recently published volume of the 1985/6 National Travel Survey[13] states that journeys of under a mile only account for 3 per cent of all personal travel mileage, and that therefore most of the main Tables in the report, which are widely quoted as definitive figures on patterns of travel, exclude these 'very short' [*sic*] journeys. As a consequence, the significance of cycling is reduced by a third—that is the proportion of journeys made over distances of less than one mile.

As has been noted, there is a considerable level of under-reporting of cycle accidents. Comparisons of casualty-rates therefore underestimate the relative danger of cycle travel and dilute the strength of those campaigning for better provision for cycling. Surprisingly, no reference to this is made in the annual published tables on road accidents.[14]

Local authorities are not obliged, or even encouraged, to isolate their expenditure on provision for cycling in their Transport Policies and Programmes as, other than in exceptional cases, this expenditure is incorporated under the heading of 'minor works' with the result that no information is kept on them.[15] Thus, there are no national records of this expenditure for analysis and there can be no regular monitoring of it. In this way, the role that cycling could play in what is seen to be the main objective of transport policy—that of achieving improved efficiency[16]—is overlooked.

Cost-benefit analysis has not been applied in the context of provision for cycling as an alternative to road building, to accommodate more traffic, even though there would appear to be a prima facie case for believing that the unit costs for providing for a cycle kilometre would be far lower than that for a car or bus-passenger kilometre—even discounting all the social and environmental elements that the current procedures exclude.

In addition, there is as yet insufficient data to calculate the savings to health, for instance, the reduction in costs on the NHS of having a fitter population if cycling were to become a more common mode of transport, as it is, for instance, in the Netherlands. Evidence examined in this report strongly suggests that a wide take-up of regular cycling could significantly improve physical fitness and would lead to a reduction of some of the considerable sums currently spent each year on treating patients for circulatory and respiratory diseases. The OPCS (Office of Population Censuses and Surveys) mortality statistics show that these diseases account for about three in five of all deaths, including one in four of the life-years lost by people who die before the age of 65. There exists too the prospect of lowering the number of people who are killed or seriously injured in accidents involving cyclists and therefore the costs of treating them. The reduction in other medical and social problems would be very likely to lead to further substantial savings as well as to healthier and longer lives.

Given the dearth of data on the cost-effectiveness—economically, socially, and environmentally—of cycling, it is surprising that the most recent figures, quoted in a written answer to a parliamentary question over two years ago,[17] indicate that only about 0.015 per cent of annual capital expenditure on roads is spent on cycling. In addition, although local authorities are encouraged to provide facilities to benefit cyclists,[18] they can obtain 50 per cent of the costs from central government only, as noted earlier, if it is aimed at increasing cyclists' safety and not simply to increase provision for cycling. Moreover, because the approved safety-related work is usually associated with new and existing trunk roads, the facilities for cyclists tend to be on cycle tracks along these roads, which are generally an inappropriate location in view of the close proximity of motor traffic.

Although the quality of the environment in terms of safety and health has been considerably lowered as traffic volumes have risen—on average, half a million more vehicles on the roads each year for the last ten years—the onus of responsibility for responding to the rising risk of injury has been steadily transferred to cyclists (and pedestrians), with increasing calls on them to exercise greater care, to wear light-coloured clothing and reflective sashes, and to wear helmets to avoid serious head injury.

The increase in traffic has also led to more noise and pollution, but there are no national noise surveys and very few monitoring-stations on air quality. For instance, the Netherlands has 300 times as many stations recording nitrogen oxide as does the UK. Instead, again, cyclists are having to 'choose' to wear smog masks to filter out some of the damaging by-products from motor-vehicle exhausts, which not only stay suspended in the air for some time before settling, but are also often expelled from the exhaust-pipes of poorly maintained engines. The great majority of the pipes are at the rear of vehicles on their left-side, that is in the direction closest to where most cyclists are riding. As has been seen, the effect of some of the emissions are harmful to health, while others are simply distasteful and can be literally sickening.

Statistics on road accidents indicate that the speeds at which vehicles are allowed to travel are set too high and are poorly enforced. Indeed, it has been calculated that the number of drivers found guilty of speeding offences each year is equivalent to one prosecution for every 700,000 kilometres travelled, that is an average of about once in a lifetime of motoring.[19] Even when motorists are caught exceeding the limit—statistically a chance of less than once in a lifetime of driving—they simply gain three or four of the twelve penalty points allowed over a period of three years.[20]

The oversight of the role that bicycles could play in transport policy is perhaps most apparent in the lack of attention paid to children's independent mobility. Not only is their level of ownership of this preferred mode, which is ideally matched to their needs, very high, but their use of them is extraordinarily low. Recent surveys in schools in different areas of England has recorded the ownership of cycles among junior schoolchildren at 90 per cent, but only 1 per cent use them to travel to school.[21] The oversight reflects the priority given to adults' increasingly car-dependent patterns of activity.

Planning for cycling

Three sets of practical measures can improve the prospects for cycling. The first entails reducing the need for motorized travel—with all its attendant unpleasant consequences. The second requires the encouragement of personal travel in ways which incur the lowest costs for the health and welfare of the community. The third is concerned with minimizing the adverse impacts on health of motorized travel and our current transport system. Accidents, pollution, noise and vibration, stress and anxiety, danger, loss of land and planning blight, and severance of communities by roads have all been identified as ways in which our current transport system damages the public health.[22] The movement of cycling from its peripheral position in transport policy would make a significant contribution to reducing such adverse effects of the transport system.

Government can take a much more positive role in using all the means at its disposal actively to promote cycling rather than treating it as a marginal form of transport. However, a critical factor influencing perception of the significance of this role is that the organization of government departments does not lend itself to take advantage of the mutually supportive and synergistic role that cycling could play in pursuit of their individual policy objectives. Their activities need to be co-ordinated so that cycling can be promoted as a means of travel and as a means of lowering road congestion—Department of Transport; as a means of health promotion—Department of Health; as a means of conserving fossil fuels—Department of Energy; and as a means of reducing carbon monoxide and other damaging gaseous emissions from motor vehicles—Department of the Environment. The most effective way for central government to promote cycling without it leading to an increase in serious injuries is through broad transport policies which promote alternatives to motor-vehicle travel, discouraging car use. In this way, more people will be able to choose to cycle rather than drive, and the conditions in which people cycle will be less threatened by traffic.

Cyclists vary in the types of route they are prepared to use, often depending on their level of experience. Cycle routes clearly need to offer advantages over other transport modes in terms of such key factors as directness, continuity, safety, comfort, speed, quality of road surface, and attractiveness of surroundings. Local authorities have the main responsibility for this. They can be encouraged to provide well-maintained cycle networks, free of pot-holes, with junction and signal facilities giving cyclists priority over other traffic. It should be noted that the potential accident savings from separating cyclists from other traffic can be negated by poor design of junctions of cycle paths and roads.

Although the development of cycle routes along back streets can be important, the routes should be near shops and other facilities which cyclists are likely to use, with good cycle-parking stands, such as Sheffield racks, for security. In planning such cycle routes it should be borne in mind that cyclists on isolated cycle tracks may be vulnerable to attack. Cycle facilities need to be integrated with other aspects of traffic management and highway design, for example, exempting cyclists from one-way measures and giving them priority in urban centres. Ideally, cyclists should have easy access to exclusive cycle routes. For instance, Delft in the Netherlands has now made provision for cyclists so that no one is more than 150 metres from such a route.[23] In the UK it is often not practicable to develop exclusive cycle routes, especially in older urban areas. Such exclusive cycle routes should form part of an integrated road-safety policy including traffic-calming techniques, special junction arrangements, and other measures to reduce motor-traffic speeds and make ordinary roads and streets safer for cyclists to use.

Government could raise its standards on motor-traffic noise and pollution, and of course properly enforce them. It could broadcast smog warnings on those days when it is advisable to avoid breathing of highly polluted air. Local authorities could be required by central government to appoint at least one officer whose prime function was to look after the interests of cyclists and to detail within their TPPs (Transport Policies and Programmes) their intentions with regard to investment in cycle networks and parking for cyclists, as well as for cycling safety. Local authorities and industry could give cycle-mileage allowances, as does the National Health Service and several London boroughs, or company bicycles, as do some Swiss organizations.[24] Employers should also be encouraged to provide facilities for employees such as showers, lockers, changing-rooms, and secure cycle-storage space as outlined in the London Cycling Campaign's 'Cycle Friendly' charter for employers.[25]

The most advantageous single measure is the restriction of speed, through comprehensive, self-enforcing traffic-calming measures, to reduce the risk of serious injury by allowing drivers more time to take averting action.[26] This is essential where cyclists have to share road-space with motor vehicles, and, where this occurs, for there to be proper enforcement of speed-limits. However, as outlined earlier, traffic-calming measures must be designed with careful regard to cyclists' safety and convenience.

Cycling should also be better integrated with public transport. Rail use and cycling—an ideal combination for fast and convenient travel—is still relatively rare in Britain, particularly when compared to other European countries such as the Netherlands. This may be partly owing to the fact that there are few stations with appropriate parking facilities such as cycle-lockers, charges are often made for the carriage of cycles, prior reservation has to be made for Inter-City travel with a bicycle, and new rolling stock has less room for carrying cycles than the old stock. Clearly, these deficiencies should be rectified for the benefit of cyclists and of British Rail which is estimated to have lost £10 million per annum (1985 prices) of potential business due to lack of services for cyclists.[27] Improved integration of public transport and cycling could lead to the promotion of cycling as a leisure pursuit. An experimental scheme initiated by the Countryside Commission involves a bus taking cyclists, and their cycles, into the Peak District.[28] This experiment will continue for the summer of 1992.

There is a need for a change in certain types of land-use planning. Given that more journeys are made by cycle in urban settlements such as York, Hull, Cambridge, and Oxford,[29] which are relatively self-contained cities—only part of the explanation for their high cycle use is the student population in the latter two—consideration needs to be given in the planning process to encouraging forms of development such as mixed land uses which are conducive to local short distance commuting. Facilities, such as schools, shops, and leisure outlets, need to be provided at the local scale in order to minimize the distances people have to travel, thereby encouraging use of bicycles and feet and reducing dependence on cars. There should be a presumption against any proposed change that could be shown to decrease the attractions of cycling, whether in terms of increasing danger, extending the distance that has to be travelled, or other factors militating against it.

Concessions can be made more often to allow cyclists to have routes across parks and along canal towing-paths. A nation-wide programme over the last twelve years of converting disused railway lines into cycle paths by the Bristol-based charity, Sustrans, has already achieved impressive results.

Continental experience

There is a need to remove the biases in wider transport policy which encourage car use. The EC has shown considerable interest in a much-enhanced role for the bicycle. The European Parliament published a radical document in 1986 entitled *The Bicycle as a Means of Transport*, and in opening the 1989 Velo City Conference in Copenhagen, the EC Transport Commissioner expressed his determination to 'integrate cycling into the European Transport Policy Planning Process'.[30]

Much can be learned from some Continental countries which are now aiming to reduce the need for new road investment, treating their towns as 30 kph zones, and are trying to make drivers pay for the hidden costs of motor-vehicle use. In this country, attempts to accommodate increases in traffic by road building still continue, and the practice of subsidizing travel through the provision of company cars continues to exist on a major scale; up to £3.5 billion annually, according to latest estimates.[31]

There are of course cultural, topographical, and other factors that explain some of the differences in the extent of cycling. The policies and practices of countries such as the Netherlands and Denmark suggest that their high use of cycles is accounted for at least as much by a policy decision on making proper provision of networks for cyclists as it is by their largely flat terrain. The Netherlands allocates 10 per cent of its capital-spending on roads to cycle facilities, and by 1986 had an impressive network of 13,500 kilometres of cycle paths.[32]

It is worth noting too that one of the European countries which has most strongly committed itself to reducing car use and increasing cycle use is Switzerland, which is somewhat surprising in view of its mountainous terrain. Sweden and West Germany have also been investing significant resources in the provision of cycle facilities and the promotion of cycling. Particularly impressive increases in cycling have been achieved in cities such as Freiburg in Germany, where enlightened policies on cycle provision have been developed in parallel with those on public transport.

Cyclists in these countries have also benefited from major programmes of traffic-calming which, by lowering vehicle speeds and reducing the differential speeds between motorized and non-motorized traffic, have led to marked improvements through lowering the risk of serious injury in road accidents. The safety of cyclists in these countries is also aided by the fact that many drivers are also cyclists and are thus able to anticipate problems from a cyclist's viewpoint.

It is not surprising that in a major study covering policy on and provision for cycling in member states of the European Community, conditions for cycling in the UK were reported as being the worst in Europe except for Belgium.[33] Riding a bicycle was reported as being less comfortable than using public transport only in Britain and Switzerland. The British evidently do not think too badly of their public transport; poor public transport was the least common reason given for cycling.

Public attitudes

Encouraging motorists to transfer to cycling requires more than simply making cycling attractive in a physical way. In countries with radical policies on cycling, it is recognized that more has to be done to stimulate cycle use. There are psychological aspects to take into account. These are difficult to deal with: people are often emotionally attached to their cars and like driving because, among other things, it gives them a status which is not conferred on them by other means of transport.

Influencing attitudes and feelings on issues such as this is extremely difficult. However, in the new town of Houten in the Netherlands, planners have tried to improve the status of cyclists by creating an environment in which they feel important. They are seen by everybody on the squares, on the boulevards, and on the main streets, while car users have to move from small residential streets to an outer ring road beyond the limits of the town and are largely invisible to the inhabitants.[34]

Whilst possibilities in Britain for planning new settlements on this model are rare, some of Houten's planning concepts, if they prove successful, could be modified for existing towns and cities in this country. Once the ethos of cycling is established, it does seem to override anti-cycling attitudes. It may well be that the tradition that conditions attitudes is nurtured both by the prevailing speed of the city and the range of distances that most people need to travel in their daily lives.

It is not only in the sphere of transport and planning policy that attitudes to cycling and the role that it can play need to change. It is apparent in the lack of interest shown to cycling in publications in the sphere of health promotion and by bodies whose terms of reference directly or indirectly cover health. In a report from an independent multi-disciplinary committee developing a future strategy for the nation's health, no mention is made of cycling in the chapter on promoting physical and mental health.[35] The only references to cycling are in the context of reducing accidents. Similarly, a major publication on a study of health and life-styles makes no mention of cycling.[36]

In a description of its 'health promotion strategy' which is aimed at linking the health issue with environmental and ecological issues, the World Health Organization highlights the range of government portfolios involved in promoting equity and health,[37] but transport is not included, suggesting that the consequences for health resulting from the use of different forms of transport are not being given the consideration they merit. One can only speculate that the reason for the omissions is that policy-makers feel instinctively that, because cycling is relatively dangerous in current traffic conditions, it would be inadvisable to encourage people to adopt it as a means of improving their health.

In aiming to promote active life-styles among children and adults, there appears to be some reluctance to point to the contribution that cycling can make. For instance, after noting the poor physical condition of children, 'ideal' activity programmes have been recommended consisting of warm-ups, aerobics, and skipping[38]—all exercises that are very unlikely to be maintained as regularly as those resulting from daily cycling, provided that safe provision can be made for it.

In this context the role of the medical profession in the promotion of good health is also of relevance to cycling. General practitioners, public-health physicians, health visitors, health-promotion experts, and other health professionals may all make an important contribution to the public's acceptance of cycling through dissemination of information on safe cycling and through the promotion of cycling as a simple means of improving physical fitness and health. Such educational work can be carried out by organizations like health authorities and provider units as well as individual health-care workers.

Indeed, health promotion has recently risen to the top of the political agenda with the publication of the Government document, *The Health of the Nation*.[39] The document outlines key areas for action, giving objectives and targets; of particular relevance to cycling are targets for prevention of road-traffic accidents. It is easy to see how cycling could play an even greater role in Government targets for increasing physical fitness, reducing coronary heart disease, and improving the general environment if steps were taken to improve current levels of safety. In fact cycling is mentioned in the document, albeit only in the context of being an appropriate means of vigorous exercise.

The Public Health Alliance, an independent voluntary association bringing together individuals and organizations committed to public health, has undertaken an in-depth examination of transport as a public-health issue.[40] Cycling is clearly identified as having a primary role in attaining the four main objectives identified for the development of a healthy transport system: to ensure access to facilities and people to meet social and economic needs for all members of society; to encourage journeys to be made by those modes which are least damaging to public health; to minimize the health-damaging consequence of each mode of travel; and to minimize damage to the environment. The Child Accident Prevention Trust, whilst having no formal policy or position on the subject, states that it would recommend cycling for children 'in a limited area', as a means of enabling children to grow into healthy adults, though it warns of the need for safe roads and the use by cyclists of safety equipment such as helmets and visibility aids.

Although not concerned specifically with promoting health, the Sports Council recognizes the benefit of cycling in its work and fully endorses the aims and objectives of a number of the national cycling bodies. Meeting the objectives of promoting sport and maintaining health through the medium of cycling on a routine basis on the daily journey to school or work does feature in some of its public information, published in association with the Health Education Authority.[41]

In this context, it is noteworthy that the National Curriculum requires that children be made aware that exercise promotes well-being and improves bodily health.[42] But time-constraints in the school limit opportunities for practical application of this knowledge through the medium of PE, and the unsafe traffic environment limits one of the most straightforward areas of application that most children could otherwise adopt, namely cycling to and from school. The Royal College of Nursing has addressed this issue in its recently published *Manifesto for Health*. Concern over the high levels of child road-traffic casualties has led the RCN to the conclusion that 'road safety, forming part of education to promote health, should form part of the school curriculum'. The RCN have also called for more cycle lanes and more pedestrian-only areas, especially in places used frequently by children.[43]

There are differing views among those with a more direct involvement in lobbying for changes in transport policy and in making provision for these changes. Some of those who are responsible for and have been improving cycle facilities oppose encouraging cycling in cities because of the danger.[44] Even official bodies concerned with transport do not necessarily acknowledge the existence of cycling as a transport mode: a survey of drivers' views on transport alternatives did not refer to cycling, but instead focused on cars and public transport, reflecting what for most are the only visible alternative modes.[45]

On the other hand, Friends of the Earth and Transport 2000—national bodies lobbying for improved transport—see cycling as a vital part of an environmentally friendly society and, in their general campaigns, advocate policies to make cycling pleasant and safer. It is clear, however, that bodies such as these have little influence on government policy compared with that of motor manufacturers, motoring organizations, road-builders, and the oil industry. It should also not be forgotten that the government itself stands to lose tax revenues if there is a substantial reduction in motor-vehicle use.

Although, generally speaking, the public image of the bicycle as presented by media and institutions has rendered it largely invisible or irrelevant, there are signs that this is changing. A recent survey found that three-quarters of respondents were strongly or slightly in favour of alleviating traffic problems by providing more cycle lanes (and pedestrianized streets), even if it might mean less road-space for cars and reduced traffic speed.[46] Half of the respondents thought these measures should be taken immediately. Indeed, the profile of the bicycle was raised in a report on this survey. Travel time on commuter journeys by different methods were compared: the cyclist's journey-time was second-fastest, beaten only by a pre-booked taxi, with the journey-time being thirty-three minutes for the taxi and thirty-five for the cyclist, who was shown as a well-dressed, fit woman rather than a scruffy young man. Further evidence of changing attitudes was revealed in a recent Gallup survey,[47] which found that 63 per cent of motorists supported city-centre car bans and that 85 per cent felt bus, rail, and tube services should be improved, with half saying that the money should come from freezing spending on roads. More importantly, traffic-calming methods, including 20 mph speed-limits, had support from 70 per cent of drivers.

It would appear that the relatively low use of cycles in this country is largely explained by a lack of attention to cycling in public policy, insufficient pressure from bodies that should be promoting cycling as an ideal form of transport—not least because of the benefits that would ensue to the nation's health—and wholly insufficient provision for cycling. The vulnerability of cyclists to injury and the fear that this induces have led to a tacit acceptance by those with responsibility for catering for transport needs and public health to overlook the role that cycling could play in both these regards. This may explain the lack of attention paid to the wide range of means whereby cycling could be significantly promoted, whilst at the same time reducing the risk of serious injury among cyclists.

CHAPTER TEN

Life-years lost versus life-years gained

Public-policy decisions involving cycling have been developed on the assumption that cycling is a dangerous activity likely to result in loss of life or severe injury. Nevertheless, studies indicate that there are benefits to those undertaking regular exercise, such as cycling, through improved health, fitness, and possibly longevity. In order to extend further the arguments outlined in this document for a wider uptake of cycling and higher priority for cycling within public policy, it would be beneficial if comparisons could be drawn between life-years lost through cycling accidents and life-years gained through improved health and fitness. In this way, current attitudes could perhaps be reversed and cycling could be afforded the much higher priority that it deserves within our current transport, environment, and health policies.

A fairly accurate measure of the total life-years lost through fatal cycle accidents in 1989—the most recent year for which figures are available—can be made by use of data on the life-expectancies of the cyclists at their age of death, that is how many further years they would have been expected to live had they not been involved in a fatal cycling accident. Table 10.1 shows that in 1989 there were 294 fatalities resulting in a total of 11,324 life-years lost.

It is not only through fatal cycle accidents that life-years are lost, and an estimation is needed of the life-years lost by cyclists seriously injured in road accidents. In attempting to gain some approximation of this latter figure, it should be noted that an individual suffering 'serious injury', as used in the Stats 19 police reports on road accidents, is defined as a hospital in-patient involving at least one night's stay. Treatment during this stay can vary widely, for instance, from obser-

Table 10.1 Life-expectancy of UK cyclists killed in road accidents, 1989

Age/age-group (years)	Number of fatalities	Life-expectancy (years)	Total life-years lost
3	1	70.5	70
4	1	69.5	69
5	1	68.5	68
6	2	67.5	135
7	3	66.6	200
8	2	65.7	131
9	4	64.7	259
10	6	63.7	382
11	5	62.7	314
12	11	61.7	679
13	11	60.7	668
14	15	59.7	896
15	11	58.7	646
16–19	27	56.2	1,519
20–4	21	53.5	1,122
25–9	15	48.6	729
30–4	12	43.7	525
35–9	12	38.9	467
40–4	15	34.2	513
45–9	12	29.6	355
50–4	18	25.2	453
55–9	8	21.0	168
60–4	18	17.2	309
65–9	17	13.7	233
70+	45	9.2	414
TOTAL	293		11,324

Note: Life-expectancy in years is taken from the mid-point of the age band.
Sources: Department of Transport, *Road Accidents Great Britain: The Casualty Report* (HMSO, London, 1990); Central Statistical Office, *Annual Abstract of Statistics* (HMSO, London, 1990), Table 2.23.

vation to ensure that the patient has not suffered concussion to attending to an injury which is so severe that the length and quality of life are seriously curtailed and there is the prospect of long-term disability.

During the course of the preparation of this report, no evidence has been found of longitudinal follow-up surveys of people seriously injured in road accidents from which an average figure of reduced life-

Table 10.2 Length of stay in Scottish hospitals of cyclists seriously injured in road accidents, 1983 (%)

Length of stay in days							
0	1	2	3	4–10	11–30	31–100	101–365
3.9	35.3	17.7	8.5	16.6	8.5	6.7	0.0

Source: R. J. Tunbridge, *The Use of Linked Transport–Health Road Casualty Data*, Research Report 96 (Transport and Road Research Laboratory, Crowthorne, 1987).

expectancy could be obtained, and no medical experts have been prepared to estimate this figure. However, there are data available on the length of stay in hospitals of people seriously injured in road accidents. Table 10.2 shows the distribution for cyclists according to the number of days they spent in hospital, from which it can be seen that the most frequent length of stay was less than two days.

Such a relatively short stay is reflected in another measure of the severity of cyclists' injuries involving treatment as an in-patient. Table 10.3 is set out according to the distribution of serious injuries on the MAIS measure (Maximum Abbreviated Injury Scale), from five surveys which isolated cyclists as a separate class of road-user. The Table shows that very few injuries indeed were so critical as to be life-threatening, with the majority of those cyclists studied suffering 'moderate' injury.

Data from these studies indicate that the level of injury suffered by cyclists involved in non-fatal accidents, as estimated by their length of stay as a hospital in-patient, is not so severe as to make a significant contribution to the total life-years lost through the fatal cycle accidents alone. During 1989 levels of injury and accident to cyclists can therefore be represented by the 11,324 life-years calculated as having been lost.

Unfortunately, it is not possible to establish such quantifiable evidence for life-years gained, although certain studies have indicated an increase in longevity for those participating in regular exercise, such as cycling. Many factors influence an individual's level of health and fitness, and longevity may not give an indication of improvements to quality rather than quantity of life. There are, therefore, very obvious barriers to any attempts to quantify the health-and-fitness

113

Table 10.3 Cyclists treated as in-patients following a road accident, according to injury severity (%)

Survey	Category of Maximum Abbreviated Injury Scale (MAIS)					
	0–1	2	3	4	5	6
Tunbridge 1980	7.6	77.0	14.4	1.0	—	—
1981	6.9	78.2	14.2	0.7	—	—
1982	10.0	71.8	15.5	2.3	0.4	—
1983	9.9	74.2	15.2	0.7	—	—
James (1983–87)	11.0	68.0	18.0		3 (scale 4–6)	

Note: MAIS classification: 0 = uninjured; 1 = minor; 2 = moderate; 3 = serious; 4 = severe; 5 = critical; 6 = maximum.

Sources: R. J. Tunbridge, *The Use of Linked Transport–Health Road Casualty Data*, Research Report 96 (Transport and Road Research Laboratory, Crowthorne, 1987); H. F. James *et al.*, *A Preliminary Report on the Distribution of Injury Severity in Serious Road Accident Casualties*, Working Paper WP/RUS/96 (Transport and Road Research Laboratory, Crowthorne, 1990)—figures are for 1983–7 projected to 1988.

benefits of cycling by means of an increase in life-years, in order to relate this to the more quantifiable life-years lost through accidents.

However, many studies in the UK and the US in the last ten years have explored the links between physical exercise, fitness, and health, and some have studied the relationship between levels of fitness and morbidity and mortality. A summary of the findings of such research may provide an indication of the increased longevity and improved health and fitness that could be conferred on those undertaking regular cycling. It may also demonstrate the need for further research into the long-term benefits associated specifically with cycling.

A major study in this country monitored over 9,000 civil servants, aged 45 to 64 at entry, over an average period of nine years and four months. This study found that the 9 per cent of men who reported that they often participated in vigorous sports, or did considerable amounts of cycling, or rated the pace of their regular walking as fast, experienced less than half the non-fatal and fatal coronary heart disease of the other men.[1] It is interesting to note that, in the context of this study, 'vigorous' cycling was defined as at least an hour per week in the round trip to work, or at least 25 miles of other cycling in the previous week.

In the early 1980s a study of 1,400 male factory workers aged 35 to 60 was carried out in order to examine the relationship between fitness and physical activity, and to explore some aspects of health status and attitudes to health. It established that the great majority of the workers had fitness levels low enough to be prejudicial to their health, and that only those who were involved in relatively vigorous activity appeared to have adequate fitness in this respect.[2] Functional capability and health protection in the form of lowered blood pressure and less body fat were found to be well above average for those whose lifestyles included vigorous activity. Of all physical-activity variables, cycling was found to have the strongest association with fitness, but only one in seven of the workers cycled. The study found that the order of difference in fitness in their favour was equivalent to that enjoyed by being five years younger for those who sometimes cycled, and ten years younger for those who regularly cycled. Whilst the cyclists were of course a self-selected sample whose life-style may have been explained by a greater attention to health in other ways, for instance, involving a better diet and lower levels of smoking and alcohol intake, in the light of other evidence cited in this chapter it seems likely that a significant part of the difference is accounted for by their patterns of physical exercise.

In the context of this report, it is noteworthy that 95 per cent of the respondents recognized exercise to be 'certainly or probably good for their health', though only 28 per cent took part in significant physical activity. The depth of their conviction, therefore, did not bring about a behavioural change for the majority. To some extent, this could be explained by their attitude to the range of activities necessary to maintain their fitness: a frequent response of those who did not cycle was that 'it would be nice to cycle if it was less dangerous'.[3]

The study also found that, whereas significantly more leisure-time physical activity was reported by non-manual skilled workers than semi-skilled and unskilled, cycling showed the opposite trend, with a significant bias in participation towards manual workers. Life-expectancy amongst manual workers is generally lower than other occupational groups; indeed, there is a clear inverse relationship between occupational class and rates of coronary heart disease and mortality.[4] This is in part explained by increased levels of smoking and alcohol abuse among manual workers,[5] although many other factors are also involved. Cycling is therefore particularly beneficial, as it appears to be an activity embraced by social classes with relatively poor health and high risk-factors.

Of particular interest is one study that did attempt to quantify the benefits of exercise in terms of increased longevity. The study, which explored possible links between mortality rates and longevity with the physical activity and life-styles of 17,000 Harvard alumni aged 35 to 84, found exercise to be inversely related to total mortality, particularly so in relation to death due to cardiovascular and respiratory diseases.[6] Those who did not exercise at all had a 60 per cent higher death-rate from heart attacks compared with those who exercised either moderately or more intensely—there was little difference between these two groups.

As Figure 10.1 shows, mortality-rates declined steadily as the energy expended increased, with the result that mortality-rates were 20 per cent lower in the age-group 35 to 49, and 50 per cent lower in the age-group 70 to 84 for those expending over 2,000 kcals per week—equivalent to daily cycling for 30 to 40 minutes—compared with those expending less than 500 kcals. After allowance for age and other ad-

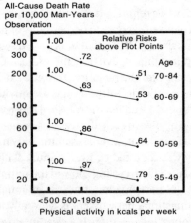

Figure 10.1 Age-specific mortality
From all causes among Harvard alumni from 1962 to 1978, according to physical activity levels.
Source: See note 6 to this chapter.

verse characteristics on health, the sedentary alumni were found to have a 31 per cent higher risk of cardiovascular mortality than the more physically active men.

By the age of 80, the weighted average increase in life-years for those expending 2,000 kcals per week, compared with those expending less than 500—a sedentary life-style—was 2.15 years, and the increase for those expending 2,000 kcals per week compared with those expending 500 to 1,999 kcals was 0.86 years. The increase in life-years among those exercising at 2,000 kcals per week was found to be equivalent to over three times that attributable to the hereditary effects of having both parents surviving beyond the age of 65. The study concluded that those who cycled 60 miles a week from the age of 35 could add two-and-a-half years to their life-expectancy.

Due to the acknowledged high levels of cycling undertaken in the Netherlands it may also prove interesting to examine data on cycle use and mortality-rates within the UK and the Netherlands. Well over a third of men and nearly two-thirds of women in the Netherlands own bicycles, and as has been seen, use of bicycles there is relatively high. Men make 25 per cent of their trips and women 32 per cent of their trips in this way, including 26 per cent and 23 per cent of the trips of men and women over the age of 65 respectively. These levels of usage are in marked contrast to those among men and women in Britain, where only 3 per cent and 2 per cent respectively of trips are made by bicycle, including less than 2 per cent of those over the age of 65.[7]

Table 10.4 shows the life-expectancy at various ages among men and women living in the UK and the Netherlands. It can be seen that, on average, in each age-group Dutch people have a higher life-expectancy for instance, at the age of 25 of one-and-a-half-years for men and two-and-a-half years for women.[8] Whilst life-expectancy is influenced by a wide range of factors, including heredity, smoking, drinking, and diet, it is not improbable to suggest that some of the difference is explained by a life-style incorporating such a significant element of exercise for a high proportion of the Dutch population.

Finally, further evidence can be provided by examination of the influence on mortality-rates of the commuting patterns of economically active people, which has been made possible for this report by

Table 10.4 Life-expectancy among males and females in the UK and the Netherlands, at various ages

	Life-expectancy in years at age			
	25	45	65	85
Male				
UK	48.4	29.3	13.4	4.5
Netherlands	49.9	30.8	14.4	4.8
Female				
UK	53.7	34.4	17.3	5.5
Netherlands	56.1	36.7	19.0	6.0

Sources: Netherlands Central Bureau of Statistics, Voorburg, the Netherlands, 1991; Central Statistical Office, *Annual Abstract of Statistics* (HMSO, London, 1990), Table 2.23.

specially commissioned Office of Population Censuses and Surveys (OPCS) tabulations. These are based on data from the record of the method of travel to work of commuters in the 1971 Census, and deaths among them during the period thereafter up to 1985. The data is presented as Standardized Mortality Ratios (SMRs), the ratio of the number of deaths observed in the study population to the number of deaths expected if it had the same rate-structure as the standard population—this ensures that spurious differences in mortality can be excluded. An SMR of 100 represents the national average. Table 10.5 shows that, compared with male commuters who travelled by methods other than by cycle in 1971, those who travelled by cycle had statistically significant lower SMRs for all causes during the fifteen years of follow-up. Though not statistically significant, the SMRs for all causes were lower too for female cycle commuters, and for ischaemic heart disease for both male and female cycle commuters.

Some of the explanation for the variation in SMRs in the Table is clearly attributable to the socio-economic circumstances of the different groups of commuters. For instance, the low rate among the men who went to work by train is likely to be related to the fact that many of them will have been living in relatively affluent households, whose members also have relatively low SMRs, in counties surrounding London. The raw data providing the figures for the Table indicate, however, that the SMRs for the cyclist are unlikely to be significantly different if the figures were adjusted for socio-economic circumstances.

It may be thought, too, that a disproportionately high number of deaths among cycle commuters would be as a result of a motor-vehicle traffic accident. But motor-vehicle traffic accidents account for only 1.4 per cent of all deaths among the commuters (with a slightly lower percentage for the cycle commuters), whereas 33.0 per cent of the deaths are accounted for by ischaemic heart disease. Whilst the proportion of cycle-commuter deaths resulting from a road accident—that is, only 12 of the 1,067 deaths from all causes—is not statistically significant, it does indicate that cycle commuters do not run an undue risk of death in a road accident, particularly if it is borne in mind that these road-accident deaths may have occurred at times other than when the cycle commuter was cycling.

In examining the data that is already available, there would seem to be an important link between lifelong exercise patterns, health, fitness, and longevity. Nevertheless, in order that the specific benefits

Table 10.5 Standardized mortality ratios (SMR) for all causes and for ischaemic heart disease, 1971–85, by means of travel to work

Means of travel	Males observed	Expected	SMR	Females observed	Expected	SMR
All causes						
Cycle	1,067	1,151.4	93*	143	155.9	92†
Car	6,876	7,495.3	92	629	747.9	84
Bus	3,882	3,290.9	118	1,433	1,332.4	108
Train	982	1,212.2	81	202	201.2	100
Motor-cycle	330	318.7	105	13	13.7	95
Walk	2,986	2,717.1	110	1,307	1,289.7	101
Ischaemic heart disease						
Cycle	398	415.1	96	19	28.7	66
Car	2,668	2,733.5	98	114	130.2	88
Bus	1,297	1,174.9	110	285	248.3	115
Train	356	435.7	82	33	35.8	92
Motor-cycle	120	113.8	105	2	2.3	88
Walk	1,013	974.7	104	243	242.8	100

Notes: * Confidence interval 87 to 98; † confidence interval 77 to 108.
Source: Office of Population Censuses and Surveys, Unpublished research (OPCS, London, 1991).

of cycling as a form of exercise may be identified, further work on the life-styles, morbidity, and mortality of cyclists is needed. In this context, evidence from the Netherlands is of particular interest and may provide the basis for further study of the mortality and morbidity of those who cycle regularly, such as the Dutch, as opposed to those who, like the British, view cycling as a marginal form of transport. In only one of the studies examined was a figure given for the proposed increase in life-years experienced by those undertaking regular exercise.[9] Similar studies with a particular focus on cycling would provide the necessary data for a true estimation of the risks of cycling when looked at in the context of benefits in health and fitness on a population basis.

Throughout this chapter we have attempted to demonstrate the benefits of cycling to the individual even in the current, largely hostile, traffic environment that led to 11,324 life-years being lost in 1989. It is obvious that any marginal difference between benefits and risks could be further reduced by making proper provision for cyclists in the form of cycle networks, bearing in mind the fact that 95 per cent of fatalities among cyclists involve a motor vehicle.[10] Evidence for minimizing the risk of accidents by the provision of cycle networks is supported by European studies in cities where such networks have been implemented. In Copenhagen, the provision of special cycling lanes reduced the risk of bicycle accidents per kilometre travelled by around 50 per cent between road junctions, but there was no reduction of accidents occurring at road junctions.[11] In a study carried out in Stockholm, similar findings indicated that, although the provision of special cycling paths reduced the risk of accidents, a limiting factor is that the paths were not separated from the ordinary traffic at road junctions, where the proportion of accidents was highest.[12]

Such improvements in provision are likely to result in an actual and perceived reduction in the risk of accident when cycling, which will facilitate and encourage a wider take-up of cycling on a regular basis by a higher proportion of the population. As has been seen, at present only about one in seven of the existing number of cycles is used several times a week.

There is a growing public consensus about the benefits to health of regular exercise. Cycling is an ideal means of sustaining a commitment to exercise throughout life, because its physical demands can be easily adjusted to levels appropriate to each individual's level of fitness and it can form part of the daily routine of travelling to school, college, or work. It is clear, therefore, that the scope for improving public health through meeting the latent demand for cycling is considerable. However, as stated earlier, rather than policy decisions being based on the proposed benefits of healthy longevity among cyclists, they have instead focused on the relatively high injury-rate among cyclists. This has no doubt contributed to discouraging people from taking up cycling, and thereby to a possible loss of life-years that could have been gained through its promotion.

Even if individuals' decisions on how to travel are taken solely from a self-interest viewpoint on how it impacts on their own health, rather than on that of the community, it may be concluded that, whilst the fatality-rate for cyclists per kilometre travelled is over eleven times the rate for motorists, compared with cycling, car travel is more deleterious to health unless the motorist is able to exercise several times a week by other means that will maintain fitness.

In this chapter a form of cost-benefit analysis of cycling has been attempted by comparing life-years lost through cycle accidents to life-years gained through regular exercise. Although a direct quantitative analysis is not possible due to a lack of conclusive data, existing evidence would suggest that, even in the current hostile traffic environment, the benefits gained from regular cycling are likely to outweigh the loss of life through cycling accidents for the current population of regular cyclists. Nevertheless, efforts should be made to enhance the safety of cyclists and improve current provision for those taking to the road.

The net benefits of cycling as an effective and accessible form of exercise should therefore be promoted vigorously by government agencies, policy-makers, health authorities, local authorities, voluntary groups, and by health professionals in a collective and individual capacity. Such commitment by these various bodies is essential in ensuring that the potential benefits of cycling, both to the individual and the wider public health, can be realized. The promotion and prioritization of cycling can make a very real contribution to improving the health of the nation.

Recommendations

Measures should be taken to reduce motor-vehicle speeds in urban areas

Two-thirds of all recorded road accidents occur in urban areas; around 95 per cent of pedestrian and 90 per cent of cycle casualties are as a result of an urban traffic accident. The critical factor is the speed of motor vehicles, since a cyclist or pedestrian hit by a vehicle travelling at more than 30 mph is likely to sustain severe injuries, whereas at speeds under 20 mph casualties are likely to be slight. For this reason, effective measures to reduce the speed of motor vehicles are essential in protecting vulnerable road-users. These include rigorous police enforcement of existing speed-limits and physical changes to road design and layout to slow down motor vehicles in urban areas. Traffic-calming measures include road-humps and speed tables, road narrowing, kerb extensions, and mini-roundabouts. Careful consideration should be given to the needs of cyclists when designing these features, for example in providing alternatives to physical obstacles such as ramps and humps in the roads and in considering road-space for cyclists when reducing the width of a carriageway. It would be unfortunate if measures to enhance the safety of cyclists by reducing the speed of motor vehicles within designated zones had the effect of discouraging cyclists from these very areas.

Cycle networks should be introduced to provide safer cycling conditions in urban areas

Local authorities should be encouraged to introduce cycle networks of various kinds according to local circumstances. These facilities may include exclusive pathways such as cycle tracks, shared cycle and pedestrian paths, cycle lanes on all-traffic roads (including contra-flow cycle lanes on one-way streets), and shared bus and cycle lanes. Such measures need to be designed with particular attention to special arrangements at junctions and main-road crossings; in addition, the approach to roundabouts should be designed to improve their safety for two-wheeled vehicles, as outlined in the recent report on cyclists and roundabouts prepared for the Cyclists' Touring Club. As well as developing new paths and networks, modifications to existing roads such as contra-flow cycle lanes and road closures with cycle exemptions should be considered. These cycle networks should cover the whole urban area, including town/city centres and cross-city routes with safe connections to surrounding countryside. All parts of the network should be well designed, with special attention to possible hazards to pedestrians and the need to protect cyclists on isolated cycle tracks who may be vulnerable to attack. Safety audits should be carried out on all such schemes to highlight any problems that may arise from junctions or crossings. Maintenance of all cycle facilities is essential. This entails maintaining a smooth surface, prompt removal of broken glass and other debris, and maintaining proper lighting and signing.

The interests of cyclists should be given more priority at every stage of the planning process for roads and transport routes

The role of the Department of Transport Regional Cycling Officers should be strengthened. These Officers need to be fully involved in all planning activities so that the needs of cyclists are considered in all trunk-road schemes, and advice can be given to local authorities in their regions about the interests of cyclists. For example, round-abouts tend to disadvantage cyclists and other two-wheeled vehicles; in considering new route design, planners should therefore consider substituting signal crossings or other measures for roundabouts where possible. Local authorities can ensure that cyclists' needs are given due attention by the judicious use of safety-audit principles and by appointing cycling co-ordinators or planning officers; these individuals would be responsible for assessing the impact of proposed schemes on the local environment, with particular attention to the safety of vulnerable road-users such as cyclists and pedestrians. Such officers would also be responsible for ensuring the intentions of the local authority, with regard to investment in cycle networks and parking for cyclists, as well as for cycling safety, are detailed in their TPPs (Transport Policies and Programmes). In general, cycling needs to be given a higher profile by government; more staff should be employed at the Department of Transport to produce practical guidance for planners and to provide effective monitoring of accidents. In addition, central government should be involved in evaluating new schemes throughout the country and disseminating the results. At present, many of the exciting initiatives to protect and promote cycling have come from local authorities, national organizations like the Royal Society for the Prevention of Accidents (RoSPA), the Cyclists' Touring Club (CTC), and local cycling or environmental pressure groups; the Government should now take a pro-active role in enhancing the safety of cyclists.

Cyclists should be made aware of their responsibilities as road-users and of their obligations under the law of the land

Cycling should be considered as a serious means of transport and, as such, cyclists, like other road-users, are subject to the Highway Code and other statutory traffic requirements. In addition to complying with all road measures such as traffic-lights and 'give way' signs, cyclists should not cycle under the influence of alcohol or drugs and are liable to financial penalty if considered unfit to cycle by a police officer. Cyclists are required by law to use lights at night; this should be rigorously enforced by the police. Other forms of making cyclists prominent should also be adopted, such as the wearing of high-visibility clothing. Cyclists should also keep their bikes in good working order by regular check-ups and servicing. Publicity and education campaigns should be developed reminding cyclists of their responsibilities for complying with the law and the common-sense measures that can be taken to make cycling safer. While adult cyclists are for the large part the victims of accidents involving other road-users, it should be noted that a small minority of accidents—five deaths in 1989—involve collisions between cyclists and pedestrians, where the latter are the vulnerable party. The Highway Code has been developed to minimize the risks of traffic casualties by all forms of road-users; cyclists must comply with the law to protect pedestrians and themselves. Local authorities should provide detailed advice for cyclists regarding responsible safe conduct on shared paths, such as the 'Cyclists' Code' produced jointly in Nottingham by the County Council and the local cycling campaign group in 1988.

Local authorities should encourage cycle use in towns by providing secure cycle parks

One important deterrent to cycling is the lack of secure public spaces in which cycles can be parked. Cycle parks should be provided at convenient central locations such as shopping centres or public libraries, and their existence should be well-publicized. Facilities should include cycle stands—such as the 'Sheffield'-type inverted U-shape rail stands—for short-term parkers and also cycle lockers for longer periods of use at appropriate places such as railway and bus stations. User-charges should be as low as is practical; local authorities should subsidize these costs in order to encourage cycling in congested urban areas. It should be noted that cycle parks are considerably more economical of space than equivalent provision for motor vehicles.

Facilities should be developed to integrate cycling more fully with other means of public transport

Cycling should be seen as complementary to other modes of transport such as buses and trains. Provision should be made for more extensive and secure cycle parking at local stations and bus stations and for safer cycle access to such interchanges. At present, there is a confusing array of conditions governing the carriage of cycles on trains; these should be made clearer to the passenger. The recent decline in arrangements for carrying bikes on trains is a cause for concern; the availability of space in the guard's van or elsewhere in the train to transport bikes should be vigorously defended. In addition, the design of future rolling stock should take into account the needs of cyclist passengers. The provision of adequate facilities for cycles on trains will become increasingly important with greater harmonization among European countries; facilities should be available throughout Europe to enable trans-boundary movement of trains and cyclists. Integration of cycling with rail travel is a good way of promoting cycling as a leisure and recreational activity; to this end, leaflets should be published promoting cycling routes linked to railway stations.

Cycling should be promoted for both utilitarian and recreational purposes by local authorities, stressing its strong health, economic, and environmental advantages

For commuter cycling it is important to stress the speed advantages of the bicycle in increasingly congested urban areas. Bicycles could be provided for staff to travel between buildings on large work-sites, in particular hospital sites. Leisure routes including local features of interest should be developed and publicized by local authorities and tourist boards in the form of maps and leaflets; these routes should be well marked by signposts. Particular attention should be paid to ensuring they are safe routes that avoid dangerous junctions. Cycle leisure routes should be developed after consultation with cyclists' groups, tourist operators, road planners, and other interested bodies such as local Groundwork Trusts. Local initiatives, such as the mass cycling event and guided rides developed in Nottinghamshire and the county-wide cycle routes promoted in Wiltshire should be further encouraged.

Local authorities should run bike-maintenance and safety courses

Evening classes should be held at regular intervals to provide cycle-repair assistance and maintenance advice. Such classes should include other features such as road-safety awareness training—

including adult cycle-training classes if possible, with some orientated to returning cyclists who have not cycled, or cycled only rarely, for many years—and the identification of cycles for security purposes by stamping numbers on the bikes by the police. In addition to the repair functions, owners of second-hand bicycles should be advised of ways of 'upgrading' their machines to British Standard levels which are currently imposed on new models. As well as evening classes, special one-day events should be arranged, such as the successful 'Dr Bike' clinics held by local cycling groups, which would combine repairs and cycle-maintenance advice with information on safety, cycle routes, and the like. Local authorities should also consider following the example of the 'Bicycle Stations' commonly found in the Netherlands, with a range of cycling facilities, including cycle hire, cycle-route information, cycle storage, and cycle-repair services.

Cycling manufacturers should assume greater responsibility for the safety of cyclists

Anecdotal evidence reveals stories of handlebars becoming detached from the bodies of bikes, brake failure, and other accidents due to poor bike design; such apparent negligence on the part of manufacturers is deplorable. Cyclists should be encouraged to report such faults and failures to consumer-protection or trading-standards officers. While British Standards protect to a certain degree the cycling consumer, it should be noted that car manufacturers have increasingly assumed responsibility for the safety and welfare of drivers and passengers; similarly, bike manufacturers should acknowledge their responsibilities for 'life and limb' of cyclists. The manner in which bicycles and cycling are advertised should be very careful not to encourage dangerous riding. Improved design in cycle lights and in the design and effectiveness of cycle helmets should be priority areas for manufacturers. More generally, manufacturers should realize that their responsibility for cycles and users of cycles does not end at the point of sale. Manufacturers could also help by improving the quality of the handbooks issued when bikes are sold. These should be different for each model and clearly and attractively illustrated.

Children and other cyclists should be encouraged to wear protective helmets

Protection from head injuries is afforded by the use of cycle helmets, although in major collisions with motor vehicles travelling at speed other injuries can assume greater significance and may indeed cause death. The argument for wearing cycle helmets is more compelling for children, as the type of accidents in which they are involved are those for which cycle helmets can provide the greatest degree of protection; that is, they do not involve collision with a motor vehicle. In addition, children are at greater risk of head injury because of their softer bone and skull structure; the 'cushioning' effect of helmets is therefore of great importance. The cost of such helmets should be subsidized by local authorities or central government; the initiatives of individual councils in introducing discount schemes for buying cycle helmets is welcomed. Government could play an important role in carrying out research to establish and improve the effectiveness of helmets and in developing improved British Standards. As the effectiveness of helmets can be greatly reduced by dropping them, manufacturers should develop a marker to indicate any damage to the helmet following an accidental knock. Adults can benefit from wearing cycle helmets; indeed, this is the most important single measure which can be taken by individual cyclists to mitigate the effects of certain kinds of road accidents. However, the wearing of helmets must be placed in the context of other means of protecting cyclists, such as motor-vehicle speed reduction, improving the conduct of drivers, and developing cycle networks and enhancing road design for the benefit of cyclists.

Cyclist training should be available for all children

This is necessary both because of the vulnerable nature of children cycling on the roads and because of the need to promote cycling and other exercise among school-age children. Figures from the Department of Transport suggest that children as a cycling population suffer disproportionately high rates of casualty, especially those aged 12 to 15 years. Equally of concern are the studies indicating low levels of vigorous physical activity among British schoolchildren. For reasons of both health and safety, road-safety practitioners and educationalists should co-operate to find ways in which cycling safety can be promoted within the national curriculum. An obvious place for inclusion of instruction on basic cycling and road-craft/safety would be within the Physical Education curriculum.

Publicity and education campaigns should be developed to raise drivers' awareness of more-vulnerable road-users, such as cyclists

While awareness of other road-users forms part of good practice in driving, attention to vulnerable groups such as cyclists and pedestrians should become a specific feature of structured driving tuition and of the driving test itself, possibly through wider dissemination of guidance such as the *Friends of the Earth Guide To Cycle Friendly Motoring*. Such awareness would include the need for cars to use indicators for the benefit of cyclists as well as other cars, and the need to avoid common faults, such as drivers turning left without making allowances for cyclists continuing along the road, or cars emerging from a side road into the path of an oncoming cyclist. Training courses for driving instructors and examiners should highlight the needs of pedestrians and cyclists, and indicate ways in which drivers of motor vehicles can protect more vulnerable road-users; where possible, those taking a driving test should be encouraged to cycle in traffic in order to experience the perspective of the cyclist. Improved information on vulnerable road-users should be provided in the Highway Code.

The accuracy and availability of accident information and statistics should be improved

Numerous studies have shown that the majority of accidents to cyclists are not reported to the police, and therefore do not appear in the Department of Transport accident statistics. The most common types of accident not to be reported involve children falling off a bicycle without another vehicle being involved. However, significant numbers of accidents that result in serious injury and do involve motor vehicles also go unreported. Police accident records should be co-ordinated with hospital accident and emergency records to provide a full and accurate picture of cycle accidents in the UK.

Random breath-testing should be introduced as a means of deterring people from driving after they have drunk excessive alcohol

It is estimated that drink-driving is responsible for about 22,000 casualties a year in the UK. Cyclists and other vulnerable road-users would benefit from any measure which was effective as a deterrent to the practice of drink-driving. The BMA has supported the call to introduce random breath-testing, whereby police officers are given complete discretion to stop drivers and request a breath-test from any motorist at any time. These police powers on breath-testing should be exercised in a targeted way by means of properly regulated spot-checks at the roadside. Following the introduction of random breath-testing in New South Wales, Australia, a 35 per-cent reduction in alcohol-related deaths and serious injuries has been achieved. Random breath-testing at designated roadside checkpoints is at present the most effective means of deterring people from driving after drinking, and should be introduced without delay.

Measures of adapting motor vehicles in the interest of cyclists should be developed

When modifying existing motor vehicles or designing new models, manufacturers should consider features which would help cyclists. One possibility is to limit all new productions to a top speed related to the national speed-limit by the use of speed-limiters; this would be of general benefit in enhancing road-safety practice. Other measures which could be considered are the modification of wing mirrors so that cyclists are more visible to drivers, and the introduction of indicators which are easier for cyclists to identify. Lorries require particular modifications in the form of front guards; bars are needed on the front of lorries as well as those currently present on the sides to prevent cyclists from falling under the wheels. One simple measure which would greatly benefit cyclists is the siting of exhaust pipes on the right-hand side of vehicles so that exhaust emissions are expelled away from cyclists, who tend to ride along the kerb-side of roads.

Cycling should be actively promoted as an environmentally friendly means of transport and an effective means of improving public health

Regular cycling, like other forms of strenuous exercise, improves the health of individuals by improving strength and endurance and contributing to lower blood pressure and weight. On a population basis, regular exercise such as cycling is associated with lower rates of mortality, especially from coronary heart disease. In addition to the health benefits to the individual and the general community, cycling has positive advantages in improving or protecting the environment. It is an energy-efficient form of transport which does not have the potential to pollute in the way that motor vehicles can and do. For these reasons, cycling should be actively promoted as a serious means of transport; the Department of Transport and local authorities should positively discriminate in favour of cyclists and pedestrians in planning transport routes and amenities and considering forms of traffic restraint. Other initiatives should be encouraged locally, in the form of special events such as the car-free day in Nottingham and the provision of facilities such as cycle parks. Local authorities and, in view of the health benefits of cycling, health authorities in particular, should be exemplary in their provision for cyclists; the London Borough of Sutton provides a mileage allowance for cyclists giving parity with motor-vehicles remuneration.

CONTACT LIST

British Cycling Federation (BCF)
36 Rockingham Road
Kettering
NORTHANTS
NN16 8HG
0536 412211

Cyclists' Touring Club (CTC)
Cotterell House
69 Meadrow
Godalming
SURREY
GU7 3HS
0483 417217

Friends of the Earth
26 - 28 Underwood Street
LONDON
N1 7JQ
071 490 1555

London Cycling Campaign (LCC)
3 Stamford Street
LONDON
SE1 9NT
071 928 7220

Royal Society for the Prevention of Accidents (RoSPA)
Cannon House
The Priory
Queensway
BIRMINGHAM
B4 6BS
021 200 2461

Transport 2000
Walkden House
10 Melton Street
LONDON
NW1 2EJ
071 388 8386

NOTES

Chapter 1

1. J. Matheson, *Participation in Sport*, Series GHS No. 17, Supplement B (Office of Population Censuses and Surveys, Social Survey Division, 1991).
2. Consumers' Association, *Which?* (Oct. 1990).
3. J. Button, *How to be Green* (Century Hutchison, 1990).
4. M. Hillman and A. Whalley, *Energy and Personal Travel: Obstacles to Conservation* (Policy Studies Institute, London, 1983).
5. M. Hillman, 'Transport and the Healthy City', in J. Ashton and L. Knight (eds.), *Proceedings of the First UK Healthy Cities Conference, University of Liverpool* (Department of Public Health, University of Liverpool, 1990); P. Draper (ed.), *Health Through Public Policy* (Merlin Press, 1991).
6. M. Hillman, 'Cycling and Health: A Policy Context', in *Proceedings of a Conference on Cycling and the Healthy City* (Friends of the Earth, London, 1990).
7. Department of Health, *The Health of the Nation: A Consultative Document for Health in England* (HMSO, London, 1991).

Chapter 2

1. R. Price and G. S. Bain, 'The Labour Force', in A. H. Halsey (ed.), *British Social Trends since 1900*, 2nd edn. (Macmillan, 1988).
2. G. K. Zipf, *Human Behaviour and the Principle of Least Effort* (Hafner Publishing Co., 1965).
3. M. Hillman, J. Adams, and J. Whitelegg, *One False Move . . . A Study of Children's Independent Mobility* (Policy Studies Institute, London, 1991).
4. Department of Transport, *National Travel Survey: 1985/86 Report—Part 1: An Analysis of Personal Travel* (HMSO, London, 1988).
5. Ibid.
6. Coronary Prevention Group, *Exercise, Heart, Health* (Coronary Prevention Group, London, 1987).

7. S. N. Blair, H. W. Kohl, R. S. Paffenbarger, *et al.*, 'Physical Fitness and All-Cause Mortality', *J. Am. Med. Assoc.* 262 (1989), 2,395–401.

8. C. Cooper, D. J. P. Barker, and C. Wickham, 'Physical Activity, Muscle Strength and Calcium Intake in Fracture of the Proximal Femur in Britain', *Br. Med. J.* 297 (1988), 1,443–6.

9. British Cycling Bureau, *Cycling—The Healthy Alternative, A Digest of 10 Reports* (British Cycling Bureau, 1978).

10. A. Hardman, *Exercise and Health: A Rationale* (Department of Physical Education and Sports Science, Loughborough University, undated).

11. Royal College of Physicians, *Medical Aspects of Exercise—Benefits and Risks* (Royal College of Physicians, London, 1991).

12. R. Read and M. Green, 'Internal Combustion and Health', *Br. Med. J.* 300 (1990), 761–2.

13. British Lung Foundation, *Breath of Life*, issue no. 5 (British Lung Foundation, undated).

14. S. Hughes, 'When the Company's Heart Misses a Beat', *Business* (Aug. 1990), 53–7.

15. British Medical Association, *Living with Risk: The British Medical Association Guide* (Penguin Books, 1990).

16. Coronary Prevention Group, *You and your Heart* (Coronary Prevention Group, London, 1989).

17. F. Giada *et al.*, 'Heparin Released Plasma Lipase Activities, Lipoprotein and Appropriate Levels in Adult Cyclists and Sedentary Men', *Int. J. Sports Med.* 9 : 4 (Aug. 1988), 270–4.

18. Coronary Prevention Group, *Exercise and your Heart* (Coronary Prevention Group, London, 1990).

19. G. Jennings *et al.*, 'The Effects of Changes in Physical Activity on Major Cardiovascular Risk Factors, Haemodynamics, Sympathetic Function, and Glucose Utilization in Man: A Controlled Study of Four Levels of Activity', *Circulation*, 73:1 (Jan. 1986), 32–40.

20. Coronary Prevention Group, *Stress and your Heart* (Coronary Prevention Group, London, 1989).

21. Ibid.

22. J. N. Morris *et al.*, 'Coronary Heart Disease and Physical Activity of Work', *Lancet*, 2 (1951), 1,053–7.

23. J. N. Morris, 'Cycling and Health', in *Proceedings of a Conference on Cycling and the Healthy City* (Friends of the Earth, London, 1990); R. S. Paffenbarger, 'Physical Activity, All-Cause Mortality, and Longevity of College Alumni', *New Engl. J. Med.* 314:10 (1986), 605–13; P. Teraslinna *et al.*, 'Relationship between Physical Fitness and Susceptibility to Cardiovascular

Disease', *Research Quarterly of the American Ass. for Health, Physical Exercise and Recreation* 39 (Oct. 1968), 746.

24. Coronary Prevention Group, *Exercise, Heart, Health*.
25. L. Sleap, 'Encouraging Habits that will Last a Lifetime', *Times Educational Supplement* (14 Feb. 1991).
26. R. Lindley, 'Passing the Fitness Test', *The Listener* (12 Mar. 1987).
27. N. Armstrong *et al.*, 'Patterns of Physical Activity among 11–16 year old British Children', *Br. Med. J.* 301 (1990).
28. Coronary Prevention Group, *You and your Heart*.
29. D. S. Sheps *et al.*, 'Production of Arrhythmia by Elevated Carboxy-haemoglobin in Patients with Coronary Artery Disease', *Ann. Intern. Med.* 113:5 (1 Sept. 1990).
30. J. N. Morris, 'Cycling and Health'.
31. H. K. Robertson, 'Heart Disease in Life-Long Cyclists', *Br. Med. J.* 24–31 (1977), 1,635–6.
32. A. J. S. Coats *et al.*, 'Effects of Physical Training in Chronic Heart Failure', *Lancet* 335 (1990), 63–6.
33. S. Rosenbaum *et al.*, 'A Survey of Heights and Weights in Great Britain', *Ann. Hum. Biol.* 12 (1985), 115–27.
34. J. Gregory *et al.*, *The Dietary and Nutritional Survey of British Adults* (HMSO, 1990).
35. J. N. Morris, 'Cycling and Health'.
36. E. A. Newsholme, 'Exercise and Obesity', in *Symposium on Exercise, Health, Medicine* (Sports Council, London, 1984).
37. P. H. Fentem, E. J. Bassey, and N. B. Turnbull, *The New Case for Exercise* (Health Education Authority, London, 1988).
38. Secondary Heads Association, *Enquiry into the Provision of Physical Education in Secondary Schools* (Secondary Heads Association, 1990).
39. Royal College of Physicians, *Medical Aspects of Exercise—Benefits and Risks*.
40. Ibid.
41. P. H. Fentem, E. J. Bassey, and N. B. Turnbull, *The New Case for Exercise* (Health Education Authority, London, 1988).
42. R. Russak, *Bicycling* 29:5 (June 1988).
43. Sports Council, *Proceedings of the Sport, Health, Psychology and Exercise Symposium, Bisham Abbey, National Sports Centre, Buckinghamshire, 26–28 October* (Health Education Authority, London, 1988).
44. D. M. W. Veale de Coverley, 'Exercise and Mental Health', *Acta. Psychiatr. Scand.* 76 (1987), 113–20.
45. N. Mutrie, 'Exercise as a Treatment for Moderate Depression in the UK

Health Service', in *Proceedings of the Sport, Health, Psychology and Exercise Symposium*.

46. J. Stephens, 'Physical Activity and Mental Health in the United States and Canada: Evidence from Four Population Surveys', *Prev. Med.* 17 (1988), 35–47.

47. H. Steinberg and E. A. Sykes, 'Introduction to Symposium on Endorphins and Behavioural Processes; Review of Literature on Endorphins and Exercise', *Pharmacol. Biochem. Behav.* 23 (1985), 857–62.

48. D. M. W. Veale de Coverley, 'Exercise and Mental Health'.

49. M. Morris *et al.*, 'Effects of Temporary Withdrawal from Regular Running', *J. Psychosom. Res.* 34:5 (1990), 493–500.

50. A. Steptoe *et al.*, 'Effects of Aerobic Conditioning on Mental Well-Being and Reactivity to Stress', in *Proceedings of the Sport, Health, Psychology and Exercise Symposium*.

51. R. Russak, *Bicycling*.

52. H. Finch and J. M. Morgan, *Attitudes to Cycling*, Transport and Road Research Laboratory Working Paper WP (HSF) 19 (Transport and Road Research Laboratory, Crowthorne, 1985).

53. J. Robertson and N. Mutrie, 'Factors in Adherence to Exercise', in *Proceedings of the Sport, Health, Psychology and Exercise Symposium*.

54. M. Hillman and A. Whalley, *Fair Play for All: A Study of Access to Sport and Informal Recreation* (Political and Economic Planning, London, 1977).

55. J. Robertson and N. Mutrie, 'Factors in Adherence to Exercise'.

56. Royal College of Physicians, *Medical Aspects of Exercise—Benefits and Risks*.

Chapter 3

1. Mintel, *Bicycles* (Mintel International Group, Sept. 1989).

2. J. M. Morgan, 'How Many Cyclists and How Many Bicycles are there in Great Britain?', unpublished Working Paper WP (TP) 36 (Transport and Road Research Laboratory, Crowthorne, 1987).

3. MORI, *Survey of the General Public* (MORI, 1990).

4. J. M. Morgan, 'How Many Cyclists . . . are there in Great Britain?'

5. M. Hillman, J. Adams, and J. Whitelegg, *One False Move . . . A Study of Children's Independent Mobility* (Policy Studies Institute, London, 1991).

6. Department of Transport, *National Travel Survey: 1985/86 Report—Part 1: An Analysis of Personal Travel* (HMSO, London, 1988).

7. J. Matheson, *Participation in Sport*, Series GHS (17) Supplement B (Office of Population Censuses and Surveys, Social Survey Division, London, 1991).

Chapter 4

1. J. A. Waldman, *Cycling in Towns: A Quantitative Investigation*, LTR1, Working Paper 3 (Department of Transport, London, Dec. 1977).

2. H. Finch and J. M. Morgan, *Attitudes to Cycling*, Transport and Road Research Laboratory, Research Report RR19 (Transport and Road Research Laboratory, Crowthorne, 1985).

3. C. Banister, 'Perceptions of Safety', Paper for a seminar organized by the Transport and Health Study Group, 23 Mar. 1988.

4. Department of Transport, *National Travel Survey: 1985/86 Report—Part 1: An Analysis of Personal Travel* (HMSO, London, 1988).

5. R. K. Herz, 'The Use of the Bicycle', *Transportation, Planning and Technology* 9 (1985), 311–28.

6. Meteorological Office, *Climatological Memorandum* 74 (Meteorological Office, London, undated).

7. C. E. P. Brooks, *The English Climate* (English University Press, 1954).

8. Meteorological Office, *Climatological Memorandum* 74.

9. Batsford, *The Cycle Tourer's Handbook* (1987).

10. Consumer's Association, *Which?* (Oct. 1990).

11. Home Office, *Criminal Statistics, England and Wales, 1989* (HMSO, London, 1990).

12. A. H. Wheeler, *Cycle Theft Update*, Department of Transport, TRRL Working Paper WP/TS/3 (Transport and Road Research Laboratory, Crowthorne, 1989).

13. Home Office, *Criminal Statistics, England and Wales, 1989*.

14. London Cycling Campaign, *Cycle Friendly Charter for Employers* (London Cycling Campaign, London, 1991).

15. T. Schmidt and J. H. Midden, 'Changing Modal Split by a Behavioural Science Approach', in *Proceedings of the Velo City 87 International Congress on Planning for the Urban Cyclist* (Netherlands Centre for Research and Contract Standardization in Civil and Traffic Engineering, Gröningen, 1987).

16. M. Hillman, J. Adams, and J. Whitelegg, *One False Move . . . A Study of Children's Independent Mobility* (Policy Studies Institute, London, 1991).

17. Ibid.

18. H. Finch and J. M. Morgan, *Attitudes to Cycling*.

19. Ibid.

20. Ibid.

21. L. Speed, 'Road User Attitudes and the Safety of Cyclists', *Cyclists' Bulletin* 44 (Friends of the Earth, London, 1988).

22. T. Bracher, *Policy and Provision for Cyclists in Europe, Report on the EC Research Project* (EC Directorate-General for Transport, Brussels, 1989).

23. W. J. Simons, 'Social Status and Position of the Bicycle in the Netherlands', *in Proceedings of the Velo City 87 International Congress on Planning for the Urban Cyclist*.

Chapter 5

1. Report on a Gallup survey, *The Times* (18 Oct. 1990).
2. British Medical Association, *Living with Risk* (Penguin Books, 1990).
3. Department of Transport, *Road Accidents Great Britain: The Casualty Report* (HMSO, London, 1990), also earlier annual volumes.
4. Department of Transport, *Transport Statistics Great Britain 1979–1989* (HMSO, London, 1990).
5. B. Preston, 'The Safety of Walking and Cycling in Different Countries', in R. D. Tolley (ed.), *The Greening of Urban Transport* (Belhaven Press, 1990).
6. Department of Transport, *National Travel Survey: 1985/86 Report—Part 1: An Analysis of Personal Travel* (HMSO, London, 1988).
7. C. S. Downing, *Pedal Cycling Accidents in Great Britain, Ways to Safer Cycling: Conference Proceedings* (Department of Transport, London, 1985).
8. J. P. Bull and B. S. Roberts, 'Road Accident Statistics—A Comparison of Police and Hospital Information', *Accid. Anal. Prev.* 5:1 (1973), 45–53; C. A. Hobbs, E. Grattan, and J. A. Hobbs, *Classification of Injury Severity by Length of Stay in Hospital*, Department of the Environment, Department of Transport, TRRL Report LR 871 (Transport and Road Research Laboratory, Crowthorne, 1979); J. B. Pedder *et al.*, 'A Study of Two-wheeled Vehicle Casualties at a City Hospital', in *Proceedings of 6th International IRCOBI Conference* (Salon de Provence, France, 8–10 Sept. 1981).
9. P. J. Mills, *Pedal Cycle Accidents—A Hospital Based Study*, TRRL 220 (Transport and Road Research Laboratory, Crowthorne, 1989).
10. M. R. Tight and O. M. J. Carsten, *Problems for Vulnerable Road Users in Great Britain* (University of Leeds, 1989).
11. C. S. Downing, *Pedal Cycling Accidents in Great Britain*.
12. Department of Transport, *Road Accidents Great Britain: The Casualty Report*.
13. Transport and Road Research Laboratory, *Hospital Study of Road Accidents* (Transport and Road Research Laboratory, Crowthorne, 1984/5); M. R. Tight and O. M. J. Carsten, *Problems for Vulnerable Road Users in Great Britain*.
14. C. S. Downing, *Pedal Cycling Accidents in Great Britain*.
15. G. Maycock and R. D. Hall, *Accidents at 4-arm Roundabouts*, Department of the Environment, Department of Transport, TRRL Report LR 1120 (Transport and Road Research Laboratory, Crowthorne, 1984).

16. R. R. Henson, *Cycling Safety at Junctions* (University of Salford, 1989).
17. Cyclists' Touring Club, *Cyclists and Roundabouts—A Review of the Literature, a Report for the Cyclists' Touring Club by Allot & Lomax, Consulting Engineers* (Cyclists' Touring Club, Godalming, 1991).
18. J. P. Bull and B. S. Roberts, 'Road Accident Statistics'.
19. S. M. Watkins, *Cycling Accidents, Final Report of a Survey of Cycling Accidents among Cyclists' Touring Club Members* (Cyclists' Touring Club, Godalming, 1984).
20. British Medical Association, *The British Medical Association Guide to Alcohol and Accidents* (British Medical Association, June 1989).
21. M. R. Tight and O. M. J. Carsten, *Problems for Vulnerable Road Users in Great Britain.*
22. Department of Transport, *Road Accidents Great Britain: The Casualty Report.*
23. D. J. Begg *et al.*, 'Bicycle Road Crashes During the Fourteenth and Fifteenth Years of Life', *N.Z. Med. J.* 104 (1991), 60–1; M. G. Lind and S. Wollen, 'Bicycle Accidents', *Acta. Chir. Scand. Supp.* 531 (1986); P. J. Mills, *Pedal Cycle Accidents—A Hospital based study.*
24. R. S. Thompson *et al.*, 'A Case-control Study of the Effectiveness of Bicycle Safety Helmets', *N. Engl. J. Med.* 320 (1989), 1,361–7.
25. J. Nixon *et al.*, 'Bicycle accidents in childhood', *Br. Med. J.* 294 (1987), 1,267–9.
26. P. J. Mills, *Pedal Cycle Accidents—A Hospital Based Study.*
27. J. Franklin and H. McClintock, 'Campaigning for what?', *New Cyclist* (Autumn, 1989).
28. Friends of the Earth, *Pro-Bike: A Cycling Policy for the 1990s* (Friends of the Earth, London, undated).

Chapter 6

1. J. McCormick, *Acid Earth* (World Wildlife Fund/Earthscan, 1989).
2. C. Holman, *Air Pollution and Health* (Friends of the Earth, London, 1989).
3. World Health Organization, *Air Quality Guidelines for Europe*, WHO Regional Publications, European Series 23 (World Health Organization, Copenhagen, 1987).
4. London Scientific Services, *London Air Pollution Monitoring Network—4th Annual Report* (London Scientific Services, London, 1990).
5. World Health Organization, *Air Quality Guidelines for Europe.*
6. Ibid.

7. J. Kagawa, 'Respiratory Effects of 2 Hour Exposure to 1ppm NO_2 in Normal Subjects', *Env. Res.* 27 (1982), 485–90.

8. C. Holman, *Air Pollution and Health*.

9. London Scientific Services, *London Air Pollution Monitoring Network—3rd Annual Report* (London Scientific Services, London, 1989).

10. C. Holman, *Air Pollution and Health*.

11. British Medical Journal, 'Internal Combustion and Health', *Br. Med. J.* 300 (1990), 761–2.

12. J. R. Goldsmith and J. A. Nadel, 'Experimental Exposure of Human Subjects to Ozone', *J. Air. Pollut. Control Assoc.* 19 (1969), 329–31.

13. World Health Organization, *Air Quality Guidelines for Europe*.

14. Molfino *et al.*, 'Effect of Low Concentrations of Ozone on Inhaled Allergen Responses in Asthmatic Subjects', *Lancet* 338 (1991), 199–203.

15. A. J. Krupnick and W. Harrington, 'Ambient Ozone and Acute Health Effects: Evidence from Daily Data', *J. Env. Econom. Man.* 18 (1990), 1–18.

16. American Lung Association, *The Health Costs of Air Pollution* (American Lung Association, 1990).

17. World Health Organization, *Air Quality Guidelines for Europe*.

18. Ibid.

19. British Medical Journal, 'Internal Combustion and Health'.

20. Department of Transport, *Transport Statistics Great Britain 1979–89* (HMSO, London, 1990).

21. Ibid.

22. C. Holman, *Air Pollution and Health*.

23. B. C. Kleiner and J. D. Spengler, 'Carbon Monoxide Exposures of Boston Bicyclists', *Air Pollution Control Journal* 26:2 (Feb. 1976), 147–9.

24. World Health Organization, *Air Quality Guidelines for Europe*.

25. D. Sheps *et al.*, 'Production of Arrhythmias by Elevated Carboxyhaemoglobin in Patients with Coronary Artery Disease', *Ann. Intern. Med.* 113 (1990), 343–51.

26. US Department of Transportation, *A Study of the Health Effects of Bicycling in an Urban Atmosphere* (US Department of Transportation, 1977).

27. A. J. Hickman, *Personal Exposures to Carbon Monoxide and Oxides of Nitrogen* (Transport and Road Research Laboratory, Crowthorne, 1989).

28. R. Read and C. Read, 'Breathing can be Hazardous to your Health', *New Scientist* (23 Feb. 1991).

29. M. Fergusson, C. Holman, and M. Barrett, *Atmospheric Emissions from the Use of Transport in the United Kingdom*, Vol. 1 (World Wildlife Fund, Nov. 1989).

30. United Nations Economic and Social Council, *Impact on Human Health of Air Pollution in Europe* (United Nations, 1990).

31. Environmental Protection Agency, *Bicycling and Air Quality Information Document* (US Environmental Protection Agency, 1979).

32. E. Krommendijk, *Bicycle and Environment in the City: A Quantitative Study into the Environmental Effects of a Bicycle Oriented Traffic Policy* (Gröningen Institute, the Netherlands, May 1988).

33. R. E. Williams, 'Rounds on a Bicycle', *Lancet* (17 Mar. 1973).

34. R. Taylor, *Noise* (Penguin Books, 1979).

35. Department of Transport, *Transport Statistics Great Britain 1979–89.*

Chapter 7

1. Mintel, *Bicycles* (Mintel International Group, Sept. 1989).

2. M. Hillman, J. Adams, and J. Whitelegg, *One False Move . . . A Study of Children's Independent Mobility* (Policy Studies Institute, London, 1991).

3. Mintel, *Bicycles.*

4. M. D. Lowe, *The Bicycle: Vehicle for a Small Planet*, Worldwatch Paper 90 (Worldwatch Institute, Washington DC, 1989).

5. Department of Transport, *Transport Statistics Great Britain 1979–89* (HMSO, London, 1990).

6. K. Otto, *Policies to Promote the Use of Bicycles as a Means of Reducing Pollution* (Federal Environmental Agency, Berlin, West Germany, 1985).

7. R. K. Herz, 'The Use of the Bicycle', *Transportation, Planning and Technology* 9 (1985), 311–28.

8. C. Banister, 'Existing Travel Patterns: The Potential for Cycling', in *Proceedings of a Conference on Cycling and the Healthy City* (Friends of the Earth, London, 1990).

9. Department of Education, *Education Statistics* (HMSO, London, 1990).

10. M. D. Lowe, *The Bicycle: Vehicle for a Small Planet.*

Chapter 8

1. M. Wierda, 'Elementary Cycling Skills and Mental Load', *University of Gröningen Traffic Research Centre Annual Report* (University of Gröningen Traffic Research Centre, 1987).

2. M. G. Lind and S. Wollin, 'Bicycle accidents', *Acta Chir. Scand. Supp.* 531 (1986).

3. P. Wells, *The State of Maintenance of Bicycles Ridden to Primary and Middle Schools*, Transport and Road Research Laboratory Report, LR 999 (Transport and Road Research Laboratory, Crowthorne, 1981).

4. Cyclists' Touring Club, *Positive Cycling* (Cyclists' Touring Club, Godalming, undated).

5. British Medical Association, *The British Medical Association Guide to Alcohol and Accidents* (British Medical Association, June 1989).

6. Department of Transport, *Children and Roads: A Safer Way* (HMSO, London, 1990).

7. M. Bennett, B. Saunders, and C. Downing, *Evaluation of a Cycling Proficiency Training Course Using Two Behaviour Recording Methods*, TRRL Laboratory Report 890 (Transport and Road Research Laboratory, Crowthorne, 1979).

8. P. Wells, C. Downing, M. Bennett, *Comparison of On-road and Off-road Cycle Training for Children*, TRRL Laboratory Report 902 (Transport and Road Research Laboratory, Crowthorne, 1979).

9. P. Roberts, *An Evaluation of a Cycling Safety Scheme in Buckinghamshire Middle Schools* (Cranfield Institute of Technology, 1987).

10. I. Van Schagen, K. Brookhuis, and M. Wierda, 'The Development and Evaluation of Two Instructional Methods for Young Cyclists', *University of Gröningen Traffic Research Centre Annual Report* (University of Gröningen Traffic Research Centre, 1988).

11. W. Maring and I. Van Schagen, 'Age Dependence of Attitudes and Knowledge in Cyclists', *Accid. Anal. Prev.* 22:2 (1990).

12. M. Wierda, 'Elementary Cycling Skills and Mental Load'.

13. H. Boyd, 'Training England's Cyclists', *Bicycle Forum* 8 (Winter 1981/2).

14. C. Juden, *Why Wear a Helmet?* (Cyclists' Touring Club, Godalming, Jan./Feb. 1991).

15. J. Darlington, *Children and Cycling* (Hereford and Worcester County Road Safety Unit, 1976).

16. B. E. Sabey, *Planning Perspectives on Traffic Safety in the UK*, Symposium on Individual Responsibility/Joint Responsibility, 1985.

17. The National Board for Consumer Policies (Konsumet Verket), *Helmets for All* (The National Board for Consumer Policies, Stockholm, Sweden, 1989).

18. Department of Transport, *Road Accident Statistics 1989, 1990* (HMSO, London, 1990).

19. Office of Population Censuses and Surveys, *Mortality Statistics, England and Wales, Accidents and Violence*, Series DH4, 12 (Office of Population Censuses and Surveys, London, 1986).

20. P. Mills, *Accident Survey*, Transport and Road Research Laboratory Research Report, RR 220 (Transport and Road Research Laboratory, Crowthorne, 1989).

21. British Medical Association, *Boxing* (British Medical Association, London, 1984).

22. C. D. Marsden and T. J. Fowler, *Clinical Neurology*, Physiological Principles in Medicine Series (Edward Arnold, 1989).

23. R. S. Thompson, F. P. Rivara, and D. C. Thompson, 'A Case Control Study of the Effectiveness of Bicycle Safety Helmets', *N. Eng. J. Med.* 320:21 (25 May 1989), 1,362–7.

24. P. Mills, *Accident Survey*.

25. R. C. Wasserman *et al.*, 'Bicyclists, Helmets and Head Injuries: A Rider-Based Study of Helmet Use and Effectiveness', *Am. J. Public Health* 78:9 (Sept. 1988).

26. R. S. Thompson, F. P. Rivara, and D. C. Thompson, 'A Case Control Study of the Effectiveness of Bicycle Safety Helmets'.

27. M. M. Dorsch, A. J. Woodward, R. L. Somers, 'Do Bicycle Safety Helmets Reduce Severity of Head Injury in Real Crashes?' *Accid. Anal. Prev.* 19:3 (1987), 183–90.

28. P. Mills, *Accident Survey*.

29. O. G. Edholm and J. S. Weiner, *The Principles and Practice of Human Physiology* (Academic Press, London, 1981).

30. C. V. Gisolfi *et al.*, 'Effects of Wearing a Helmet on Thermal Balance while Cycling in the Heat', *The Physician and Sportsmedicine* 1 (16 Jan. 1988).

31. B. D. Weiss, 'Childhood Bicycle Injuries: What Can We Do?', *Am. J. Dis. Child.* 141 (Feb. 1987), 135–6.

32. F. Donnelly, *Cycle Standards, Conference Proceedings on Ways to Safer Cycling* (HMSO, London, 1985).

33. R. H. Jackson, 'Some Aspects of Transport-related Accidents to Children in the UK', *Transport Review* 9:3 (1989), 267–78.

34. C. Juden, *Why wear a Helmet?*

35. Municipal Review and AMA News (Aug./Sept. 1990), 143.

36. T. Wood and P. Milne, 'Head Injuries to Pedal Cyclists and the Promotion of Helmet Use in Victoria, Australia', *Accid. Anal. Prev.* 29:3 (1988), 177–85; S. Ferris, S. Roberts, and K. Condon, 'Cycle Injuries and Attitudes to Safety Helmets', *Br. J. Accid. Emergency Med.* (Dec. 1989), 4–7.

37. J. Howland *et al.*, 'Barriers to Bicycle Helmet Use among Children', *Am. J. Dis. Child.* 143 (June 1989).

38. J. D. Sargent, M. G. Peck, and M. Weitzman, 'Bicycle Mounted Child Seats—Injury Risk and Prevention', *Am. J. Dis. Child.* 142:7 (Jul. 1988), 765–7.

39. M. McCarthy, 'Cycling, Risk and Health Promotion', in *Proceedings of a*

Conference on Cycling and the Healthy City (Friends of the Earth, London, 1990).

40. A. F. Williams, 'Factors in the initiation of Bicycle–Motor Vehicle Collisions', *Am. J. Dis. Child.* 130 (1976), 370.

41. Department of Transport, *Road Accident Statistics 1989, 1990.*

42. G. R. Watts, *Pedal Cycle Lamps and Reflectors—Some Visibility Tests and Surveys,* Transport and Road Research Laboratory Report LR 1108 (Transport and Road Research Laboratory, Crowthorne, 1984).

43. R. Van der Plas, 'Cycling at Night', *Bicycle* (Nov. 1984), 18–21.

44. G. R. Watts, *Evaluation of Conspicuity Aids for Pedal Cyclists,* Transport and Road Research Laboratory Report LR 1103 (Transport and Road Research Laboratory, Crowthorne, 1984).

45. Department of Transport, *Road Accident Statistics 1989, 1990.*

46. G. R. Watts, *Pedal Cycle Lamps and Reflectors—Some Visibility Tests and Surveys.*

47. G. R. Watts, *Evaluation of Conspicuity Aids for Pedal Cyclists.*

48. Department of Transport Leaflets: *Lesson for Life, Teaching Road Safety for Parents of 1–15 Year Olds;* and *Bright Sparks: Be Safe Be Seen* (HMSO, London, 1990).

49. G. R. Watts, *Evaluation of Conspicuity Aids for Pedal Cyclists.*

50. G. R. Watts, *Pedal Cycling Braking Performance—Effects of Brake Block and Rim Design,* Transport and Road Research Laboratory Digest SR 619 (Transport and Road Research Laboratory, Crowthorne, 1980).

51. G. R. Watts, *Evaluation of Conspicuity Aids for Pedal Cyclists.*

52. J. G. U. Adams, *Risk and Freedom: The Record of Road Safety Regulation* (Transport Publishing Projects, Cardiff, 1985).

53. 'Pollutant Masks Hide Risk to City Cyclists', *New Scientist* (25 Aug. 1990), 28.

54. *London Cyclist* (Nov./Dec. 1990).

55. British Lung Foundation, *Air Pollution and the Lungs* (British Lung Foundation, London, undated).

Chapter 9

1. Department of Transport, *Transport Policies and Programme Submissions for 1991/92,* Local Authority Circular 1/90 (Department of Transport, London, Apr. 1990).

2. Department of Transport, *Children and Roads: A Safer Way* (HMSO, London, 1990).

3. J. Atkins, *Hansard,* col. 190 (24 Apr. 1990).

4. H. McClintock, 'Traffic Calming—The Cyclist's Viewpoint', in *Traffic*

Calming in Theory and Practice Conference, University of Nottingham, 24 May 1990.

5. Cyclists' Touring Club, *Traffic Calming Technical Note* (Cyclists' Touring Club, Godalming, 1991).

6. R. Chope, *Hansard*, col. 6 (22 Oct. 1990).

7. R. Chope, Letter to *The Times* (15 Nov. 1990).

8. Written answer, *Hansard*, col. 249 (25 Oct. 1990).

9. Department of Transport, *Transport: A Guide to the Department* (HMSO, London, 1990).

10. S. Skinner, *Moving America: New Directions, New Opportunities*, Policy Paper of the US Secretary of State for Transportation (1990).

11. A. Nicholls, *Annual Conference of the National Society for Clean Air*, 1990, Newcastle.

12. M. D. Lowe, *The Bicycle: Vehicle for a Small Planet*, Worldwatch Paper 90 (Worldwatch Institute, Washington DC, 1989).

13. Department of Transport, *National Travel Survey: 1985/86 Report—Part 1: An Analysis of Personal Travel* (HMSO, London, 1988).

14. Department of Transport, *Road Accidents Great Britain 1989: The Casualty Report* (HMSO, London, 1990).

15. Written answer, *Hansard*, col. 607 (31 Jan. 1991).

16. J. Rickard, *Private and Public Investment in Transport*, European Community Ministers of Transport Round Table 81 (Economic Research Centre, Brussels, 1990).

17. Written answer, *Hansard*, col. 446 (20 Jun. 1988).

18. Department of Transport, *Transport Policies and Programme Submissions for 1991/92*.

19. S. Plowden and M. Hillman, *Danger on the Road: The Needless Scourge* (Policy Studies Institute, London, 1984).

20. Ibid.

21. M. Hillman, J. Adams, and J. Whitelegg, *One False Move . . . A Study of Children's Independent Mobility* (Policy Studies Institute, London, 1991).

22. Public Health Alliance, *Health on the Move: Policies for Health Promoting Transport, The Policy Statement of the Transport and Health Study Group* (Public Health Alliance, Birmingham, 1991).

23. R. Tolley, 'Green Transport', *The Geographical Magazine* (Aug. 1988), 41–3.

24. National Economic Development Council, *Company Cars: An Interim Perspective* (National Economic Council, 1991).

25. London Cycling Campaign, *Cycle Friendly Charter for Employers* (London Cycling Campaign, London, 1991).

26. S. Plowden and M. Hillman, *Danger on the Road: The Needless Scourge.*

27. Harris Research Centre, *Cycles (and other Bulky Luggage) on Trains* (Harris Research Centre, London, 1984).

28. Transport for Leisure and the Department of Planning and Landscape, University of Manchester, *Cycle Transport Network Study: A Study Undertaken for the Countryside Commission North-West Office* (Department of Planning and Landscape, Manchester, 1991).

29. C. Banister, 'The Policy Implications of the Travel to Work Patterns for Pedestrians and Cyclists', paper given at PTRC Summer Annual Meeting, 1987.

30. K. Van Miert, 'Cycling as part of the EEC Transport and Environment Policy', in *Proceedings of the Velo City Conference*, Copenhagen, 1990.

31. Greenpeace, *Company Car Costs in the United Kingdom* (Greenpeace, London, 1991).

32. M. D. Lowe, *The Bicycle: Vehicle for a Small Planet.*

33. T. Bracher, H. Krafft-Neuhauser, and H.-P. Preusser, *Policy and Provision for Cyclists in Europe* (Commission of the European Communities, Directorate-General for Transport, Brussels, 1989).

34. R. W. Meilof, 'Town Planning, Ways to Stimulate Bicycle Use. How to Plan Urban Developments', in *Proceedings of the Velo City 87 International Congress on Planning for the Urban Cyclist* (Netherlands Centre for Research and Contract Standardization in Civil and Traffic Engineering, Gröningen, 1987).

35. A. Smith, B. Jacobson, *The Nation's Health: A Strategy for the 1990s, A Report from an Independent Multidisciplinary Committee* (King's Fund, London, 1988).

36. M. Blaxter, *Health and Lifestyles* (Tavistock/Routledge, 1990).

37. I. Kickbusch, *A Strategy for Health Promotion: A Description of the Health Promotion Programme at the Regional Office for Europe* (World Health Organization, Copenhagen, 1989).

38. L. Sleap, 'Encouraging Habits that will Last a Lifetime', *Times Educational Supplement* (14 Feb. 1991).

39. Department of Health, *The Health of the Nation: A Consultative Document for Health in England* (HMSO, London, 1991).

40. Public Health Alliance, *Health on the Move: Policies for Health Promoting Transport.*

41. Sports Council and Health Education Authority, *Exercise. Why Bother?* (Health Education Authority, London, 1990).

42. National Curriculum Council, *Curriculum Guidance 5: Health Education* (National Curriculum Council, London, 1990).

43. Royal College of Nursing, *A Manifesto for Health* (Royal College of Nursing, London, 1991).

44. B. Oldridge, 'Highway Engineering', in *Conference Proceedings on Ways to Safer Cycling* (Department of Transport, London, 1985).

45. Metropolitan Transport Research Unit, *North East London Attitudes to Traffic Restraint: Final Report* (Apr. 1990).

46. Consumers' Association, *Which?* (Oct. 1990).

47. 'Motorists Back Car Ban in Cities', *Guardian* (26 July 1991).

Chapter 10

1. J. N. Morris *et al.*, 'Exercise in Leisure Time: Coronary Attack and Death Rates', *Br. Heart J.* 63 (1991), 325–34.

2. W. Tuxworth *et al.*, 'Health, Fitness, Physical Activity and Morbidity of Middle-aged Male Factory Workers', *Br. J. Ind. Med.* 43 (1986), 733–53.

3. Ibid.

4. M. G. Marmot and M. E. McDowall, 'Mortality Decline and Widening Social Inequalities', *Lancet* 2 (1986), 274–6.

5. A. Rosengren, H. Wedel, and L. Wilhelmsen, 'Coronary Heart Disease and Mortality in Middle-aged Men from Different Occupational Classes in Sweden', *Br. Med. J.* 297 (10 Dec. 1988).

6. R. S. Paffenbarger *et al.*, 'Physical Activity, All-Cause Mortality and Longevity of College Alumni', *New Engl. J. Med.* 314:10 (1986), 605–13.

7. Department of Transport, *National Travel Survey: 1985/86 Report—Part 1: An Analysis of Personal Travel* (HMSO, London, 1988).

8. Netherlands Central Bureau of Statistics, Voorburg, the Netherlands, 1991.

9. R. S. Paffenbarger *et al.*, 'Physical Activity, All-Cause Mortality and Longevity of College Alumni'.

10. Department of Transport, *Road Accidents Great Britain: The Casualty Report* (HMSO, London, 1990).

11. N. O. Jørgensen and L. Hanstedt, *Sikkerhed for cyklister og Knallertkørere i Københavnsområdet. Sammanfattning.* Rådet for Trafiksikkerhedsforskning; Report 24 (Rådet for Trafiksikkerhedsforskning, Copenhagen, 1979).

12. M. G. Lind and S. Wollin, 'Bicycle accidents', *Act Chir. Scand. Suppl.* 531 (1986).

GLOSSARY

aerobic exercise. Exercise where the energy-demand is met by available oxygen (oxidative metabolism). This usually involves repetitive, low-intensity contractions of large muscle groups for prolonged periods as in cycling, swimming, and jogging.

airway resistance. The opposition to force offered by the airway (passage from the outer air to the lungs) to flow of respiratory gas in and out of the lungs. Used as a measure of effective lung function.

all-cause mortality. Death-rate due to any cause.

all-terrain bike (ATB). More commonly known as the 'mountain bike'. A rugged bike intended for off-road use, though popular for on-road use due to uneven road surfaces and pot-holes.

anaerobic exercise. Exercise during which anaerobic metabolism occurs as the energy requirement exceeds that which can be met by available oxygen. Found during exercise of short but intense duration, such as sprinting, sprint cycling, jumping, or press-ups.

arrhythmogenic. Strictly speaking lack of heartbeat. Arrhythmogenic is commonly used for abnormal beating of the heart.

atherosclerosis. A condition in which a combination of changes occurs in the innermost coating of the arteries consisting of accumulation of lipids (fats), complex carbohydrates, blood and blood products, fibrous tissue, and calcium deposits. This is associated with increased blood pressure and narrowing of arteries which can be blocked by clots leading to stroke and/or heart attacks.

benzene. A chemical known to cause cancer but that occurs in the air of all European cities, 80 per cent of which is due to motor-vehicle exhaust emissions. Member of the class of compounds known as Volatile Organic Compounds (VOCs).

Bicycle Moto-Cross (BMX). A bike intended for off-road use with the centre of gravity towards the rear of the cycle, enabling stunts to be performed.

bronchial responsiveness. The degree of response observed in the bronchi (the main forks and sub-branches of the windpipe that enter the lungs) due to certain stimuli, for example, the degree of constriction observed in response to allergens.

carboxyhaemoglobin. A compound formed upon contact of haemoglobin with carbon monoxide, for which it possesses 300 times greater affinity than for oxygen. Its formation in the blood reduces the amount of oxygen that can be carried. Inhalation of carbon monoxide is therefore dangerous.

cardiovascular disease. An umbrella term for diseases of the heart and blood vessels encompassing such conditions as coronary heart disease and high blood pressure.

cardiovascular mortality. Death-rate associated with disease of the heart and blood vessels.

conurbation. Large urban area formed where towns have spread and merged.

coronary heart disease. Atherosclerotic disease of the coronary arteries which surround and supply the heart, used synonymously with the term 'ischaemic heart disease'.

cost–benefit analysis. A mechanism for evaluating something's worth through examining its cost in relation to the benefits obtained. For example, how the cost of providing a new pedestrian crossing relates to the costs saved by the subsequent reduction in injuries and fatalities.

Cycleway. An educational programme to help children develop a fuller understanding of safer cycling, by combining classroom activities involving pupils discussing and solving problems with teaching them to cycle on quiet roads.

defensive cycling. A technique whereby the cyclist defers to motor vehicles to avoid danger. For example, dismounting and using a pedestrian crossing when turning right so as not to be left waiting to turn in the middle of a busy road.

fitness. Ability to carry out certain activities. Not to be confused with 'health' which can be defined as absence of illness.

forced expiratory volume. The maximum volume of air produced by forced expiration of air from the lungs. Used as a measure of lung function.

formaldehyde. Colourless gas used in solution as a preservative and disinfectant. Member of the class of compounds known as Volatile Organic Compounds (VOCs).

General Household Survey. An annual survey carried out by the Office of Population Censuses and Surveys on a sample of the population (normally 10,000 households) living in 'non-institutional' residences (that is, not prisons, nursing homes, and so on). The survey asks basic questions about family structure, employment, and health and is used by the government in planning resource-allocation.

greenhouse gases. Gases such as chlorofluorocarbons (CFCs), carbon dioxide, methane, nitrous oxide, and tropospheric ozone, which trap outgoing radiation reflected back from the earth's surface; this has the effect of warming the lower atmosphere (the 'Greenhouse effect').

haemoglobin. The complex protein molecule contained within the red blood cells which gives them their colour and by which oxygen is transported around the body.

hydrocarbons. Any organic compound consisting of hydrogen and carbon only, such as benzene. There are several hundred such compounds formed mainly as a result of incomplete combustion of organic materials, such as fossil fuels. Hydrocarbons are a subclass of the class of compounds known as Volatile Organic Compounds (VOCs).

ischaemic heart disease. Disease resulting from an insufficient blood-supply to the heart relative to its needs, usually the result of atherosclerotic disease of the blood vessels supplying the heart. Used synonymously with coronary heart disease.

life-years gained. The extra years of life gained—for example, due to lifelong participation in regular exercise—over and above the predicted life-expectancy of an individual.

life-years lost. The further years that an individual could have expected to live if they had not died prematurely. For example, the number of further years an individual would have been expected to live had he or she not been involved in a fatal cycling accident.

life-expectancy. A standard measure of the number of further years that individuals can expect to live for their given age.

longitudinal follow-up survey. A survey that is carried out to discover the effects over time of an incident or illness. For example, a survey of those suffering road-traffic accidents that follows the individual's progress to see how quality of life or eventually length of life is affected.

maximum abbreviated injury scale (MAIS). A numerical scale used to classify an individual's level of injury. The scale ranges from 0 = uninjured to 6 = maximum.

monoamine. A class of chemical compounds of which many of the important neurotransmitters (chemicals which enable transfer of nervous impulses) of the peripheral and central nervous system are members. Drugs for the treatment of various mental-health problems often elicit their effects by blocking the breakdown of monoamines.

morbidity. Disease or ill health.

mortality. Death.

mountain bike. See 'all-terrain bike'.

national cycling-proficiency scheme (NCPS). A training-scheme for young cyclists, to train children in basic cycle manœuvres, teach them the relevant sections of the Highway Code, and to encourage them to maintain their cycles in a roadworthy condition.

opioid peptides. A class of chemical compounds that act as neurotransmitters (chemicals which enable transfer of nervous impulses). Some of the receptors in the nervous system through which the drug morphine has an effect are the receptors by which the peptides also elicit their effect.

osteoporosis. A metabolic bone disease involving a reduction in bone mass to a level which may lead to fracture, especially of the spine, forearm, and hip.

photochemical oxidants. Oxidants formed due to a chemical reaction which is initiated, assisted, or accelerated by exposure to light, chiefly visible and ultraviolet. Most commonly a reaction between nitrogen oxides and certain hydrocarbons forming, for example, ozone.

photochemical smog. The phenomenon found in heavily motorized cities where reactions, particularly between nitrogen oxides and hydrocarbons, under the influence of sunlight can produce poor visibility, a brown pall in the air, eye irritation, and damage to materials and vegetation.

polycyclic aromatic hydrocarbons. A subgroup of the chemical compounds known as aromatic hydrocarbons, which are commonly found in petroleum products containing as part of their structure rings of atoms such as are found in benzene and other similar cyclic molecules. Many of such compounds have been shown to cause cancer.

safety audit. A periodic examination of the financial consequences of safety measures.

Sam Browne belt. A reflective and fluorescent strap worn around the waist and diagonally across the body to attract motorists' attention to two-wheeled-vehicle users.

Sheffield rack. An inverted 'u'-shaped bike rack to which a cycle may be secured, which is normally the preferred type of bike rack by cyclists.

single/double British summer-time. Whereby the clock would be one hour ahead of the present GMT/BST time for most of the year, giving more hours of daylight in the evening than the morning.

standardized mortality ratio (SMR). The ratio of the number of deaths observed in the study population to the number of deaths expected if it had the same rate-structure as the standard population; an SMR of 100 represents the national average.

stats 19. A form filled out by the police when attending a road-traffic accident.

The information provided on this form is used to generate Department of Transport statistics on road-traffic accidents.

stratosphere. The second-lowest level of the earth's atmosphere, approximately 8 km. to 80 km. in depth, in which temperature is fairly constant and where the ozone layer is found.

synergistic. The phenomenon in which the effect produced by two (or more) substances together is greater than the sum of the effects produced by the substances separately.

topography. The study of surface features and land forms of an area.

traffic-calming. Mechanisms intended to reduce the speed of motor vehicles; for example, speed humps.

ventricular arrhythmia. Strictly speaking, absence of ventricular beat. Arrhythmia is used synonymously with disrhythmia to mean irregularity in the rhythm of the ventricles, or pumping chambers, of the heart.

volatile organic compounds (VOCs). The name given to a class of organic compounds which evaporate easily and contribute to air pollution mainly through the production of secondary pollutants such as ozone. VOCs include the hydrocarbons and other, more complex, organic substances. Some are produced by natural processes, but motor vehicles and some industries are equally significant sources.

vulnerable road-user. A term used to describe road-users who are more susceptible to accident due to their inability to control the type of incident in which they are commonly involved, usually employed when referring to cyclists and pedestrians.

wind chill. Cooling effect of wind blowing on a surface.

INDEX